Group Music Therapy

In *Group Music Therapy* Alison Davies, Eleanor Richards and Nick Barwick bring together developments in theory and clinical practice in music therapy group work, celebrating the richness of what group analytic thinking and music therapy can offer one another. The book explores the dynamic elements of the processes that take place in group analytic therapy and group music therapy, exploring both the commonalities and the distinctive characteristics of the two modalities.

To music therapists, psychotherapists and other arts therapists, *Group Music Therapy* offers a body of knowledge and enquiry through which to understand the music therapy group process through some of the central proposals of group analysis; to group analysts it offers insight into the possibilities of non-verbal communication through improvised music and, more widely, invites thought in musical terms about the nature of events and exchanges in a therapy group. Links are made with group analytic theory as well as with other associated theoretical traditions, such as attachment theory and theories of early infant development. The book explores the history of group music therapy and the history of group analysis, looking at both core concepts and more recent developments. Attention is also given to developmental issues, drawing upon theories of infant development and attachment theory, and clinical vignettes drawn from music therapy practice with a wide range of patient groups illustrate these ideas. The book concludes with a discussion of the possibilities of co-therapy and other collaborative working and of the value of experiential groups in training.

Group Music Therapy will be a key text for clinicians and students seeking to expand their theoretical thinking and enrich their practice, and offers a grounding in group analytic ideas to professionals in other disciplines considering referrals to group work.

Alison Davies trained as a music therapist and a psychoanalytic psychotherapist. She has worked in the NHS and in private practice and has run groups for music therapy trainees at Anglia Ruskin University, Cambridge, and the Guildhall School of Music and Drama, London. She has also taught and run groups for the Philadelphia Association psychotherapy training.

Eleanor Richards is a senior lecturer in music therapy at Anglia Ruskin University, Cambridge, and a psychoanalytic psychotherapist and supervisor in private practice. She has a longstanding interest in group work and is involved in the development of music therapy training and practice in India.

Nick Barwick is a group analyst who has conducted groups in the NHS, higher education and private practice. He is Head of Counselling at the Guildhall School of Music and Drama, London, where he also teaches on the MA in Music Therapy. He is immediate past editor of the journal *Psychodynamic Practice*.

Group Music Therapy

A group analytic approach

Alison Davies, Eleanor Richards and Nick Barwick

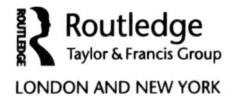

Routledge
Taylor & Francis Group

LONDON AND NEW YORK

First published 2015
by Routledge
27 Church Road, Hove, East Sussex, BN3 2FA

and by Routledge
711 Third Avenue, New York, NY 10017

Routledge is an imprint of the Taylor & Francis Group, an informa business

© 2015 Alison Davies, Eleanor Richards and Nick Barwick

The right of Alison Davies, Eleanor Richards and Nick Barwick to be identified as authors of this work has been asserted by them in accordance with sections 77 and 78 of the Copyright, Designs and Patents Act 1988.

All rights reserved. No part of this book may be reprinted or reproduced or utilised in any form or by any electronic, mechanical, or other means, now known or hereafter invented, including photocopying and recording, or in any information storage or retrieval system, without permission in writing from the publishers.

Trademark notice: Product or corporate names may be trademarks or registered trademarks, and are used only for identification and explanation without intent to infringe.

British Library Cataloguing in Publication Data
A catalogue record for this book is available from the British Library

Library of Congress Cataloging in Publication Data
Davies, Alison, 1943-
  Group music therapy : a group analytic approach/Alison Davies, Eleanor Richards and Nick Barwick.
     p. cm.
  Includes bibliographical references.
  1. Music therapy. 2. Group psychotherapy. I. Richards, Eleanor (Eleanor Gurney) II. Barwick, Nick, 1959– III. Title.
  ML3920.D27 2014
  615.8'5154—dc23
                                                    2014012895

ISBN: 978-0-415-66592-6 (hbk)
ISBN: 978-0-415-66594-0 (pbk)
ISBN: 978-1-315-75257-0 (ebk)

Typeset in Times New Roman
by RefineCatch Limited, Bungay, Suffolk

Printed and bound in Great Britain by
TJ International Ltd, Padstow, Cornwall

Contents

Notes on contributors vii
Foreword ix
BILL LINTOTT
Preface xii
ELEANOR RICHARDS
Acknowledgements xiv

PART 1
Group music therapy: Historical perspectives 1

1 **Music therapy and the development of group work** 3
   ALISON DAVIES

2 **The development of group work in music therapy in the UK** 12
   HELEN ODELL-MILLER IN CONVERSATION WITH ELEANOR RICHARDS

PART 2
Group therapy: A group analytic perspective 25

3 **Core concepts in group analysis: What goes on in groups? (Part 1)** 27
   NICK BARWICK

4 **Core concepts in group analysis: What goes on in groups? (Part 2)** 36
   NICK BARWICK

5 Core concepts in group analysis: What does the conductor do?   48
NICK BARWICK

6 Developments in group analysis: The mother approach   67
NICK BARWICK

7 Developments in group analysis: The 'other' approach   78
NICK BARWICK

PART 3
Group music therapy: Developmental perspectives   89

8 Early years: Experiences with others   91
ALISON DAVIES

9 Music, attachment and the group: Mainly theory   100
ELEANOR RICHARDS

10 Music, attachment and the group: Mainly practice   109
ELEANOR RICHARDS

PART 4
Group music therapy: Clinical perspectives   119

11 Clinical vignettes   121

12 Co-therapy and working with others   139
ALISON DAVIES

13 Experiential groups on music therapy trainings   149
ALISON DAVIES

References   163
Index   176

Contributors

Luke Annesley graduated in Music and Ethnomusicology from Cambridge University and then worked as a freelance saxophonist/clarinettist, teacher and workshop leader. He qualified as a music therapist in 2008. After spending a year as a therapist for the charity Kids Company, he continues to work for Oxleas Music Therapy Service (NHS) and with CAMHS and 'Housing for Women' on a project focusing on children who have been exposed to domestic violence. He is a visiting lecturer in music therapy at City University, London.

Nick Barwick is a group analyst who has conducted groups in the NHS, higher education and private practice. He is Head of Counselling at the Guildhall School of Music and Drama, London, where he also teaches on the MA in Music Therapy. Both writer and musician, he has a particular interest in helping people overcome creative blocks/inhibitions. He is immediate past editor of the journal *Psychodynamic Practice*.

Catherine Carr is a music therapist and NIHR Clinical Doctoral Fellow at Queen Mary University of London, and research supervisor and lecturer for the MA in music therapy at the Guildhall School of Music and Drama. Her interests are in music therapy and adult mental health, including acute inpatient care and post-traumatic stress disorder.

Stella Compton Dickinson is a Fellow and Member of the Institute of Mental Health, Nottingham, and an Honorary Researcher at the Institute of Psychiatry, London. She held the posts of Head of Arts Therapies and Clinical Research Lead at Rampton National High Secure Hospital from 2001–2013. She is an accredited cognitive analytic therapist and supervisor, an HPCP registered music therapist, and a researcher and consultant lecturer. She has presented her work internationally. She continues to be active in her first career as a professional oboist and teacher.

Alison Davies trained as a music therapist at Roehampton Institute, London, and as a psychoanalytic psychotherapist with the Philadelphia Association. She has run music therapy groups and talking groups in varied settings for over 20 years and has a particular interest in mental health. She has been involved in training music therapists at the Guildhall School of Music and Drama and at Anglia Ruskin University. She has contributed to various publications and spoken at international conferences.

Karen Gold is a music therapist working with older people with dementia, children and young people, and mothers with post-natal depression and their babies. She is training as a psychoanalytic psychotherapist. The groups described in her contribution here took place in NHS out-patient settings.

Alison Levinge has a lifelong interest in early attachment issues, which found expression through her previous position as a trainer of music therapists and continues through her activity as a clinician and writer. Her initial research was into aspects of Winnicott's ideas; that gave rise to her particular interest in using music therapy with mothers and their babies together. Her current clinical practice is with children and their families affected by life threatening illness or bereavement. She also lectures internationally and has published widely.

Eleanor Richards is a senior lecturer in music therapy at Anglia Ruskin University, Cambridge, and a psychoanalytic psychotherapist and supervisor in private practice. She has a longstanding interest in group work, especially with people (such as some in the learning disabled community) who may find flexible interaction particularly difficult. She is co-editor (with Alison Davies) of *Music Therapy and Group Work* (2002) and has contributed to a range of publications and international conferences. She is involved in the development of music therapy training and practice in India.

Ann Sloboda is Head of Music Therapy at the Guildhall School of Music and Drama, London. She has worked as a music therapist in the NHS for many years in acute and forensic psychiatry settings, and has headed a team of arts therapists. She trained as a psychoanalyst at the British Institute of Psychoanalysis and qualified in 2012.

Foreword

Bill Lintott

In this book three gifted therapists describe the development and practice of group analysis and music therapy, drawing on their own experience and the experiences of others to give a vivid account of this work. Their approach to therapy values highly the insights of all group members, whatever they may bring. In a world of controls and authorities and expert knowledge, where human technical ability has never been greater, this is precious.

More and more we rely on the cleverness of others to solve problems, often for good reason. Experts provide solutions. Much of their knowledge and skill brings huge benefits. But how they do this is often beyond our understanding. Should we always trust those with expert knowledge to use it well or wisely? Unquestioning reliance on processes we do not know about or cannot understand places enormous power in the hands of others – the power, for instance, to pry into people's lives. Modern technology has made possible widespread intrusion, which is largely carried on in secret. The devices in our pockets can track our movements and contacts at all times. No child born today will ever experience genuine privacy or self-reliant solitude. Little more than a lifetime ago, explorers could be cut off from all contact with the rest of the world for years at a time, reliant on themselves alone for their very survival; now every corner of the earth is watched over by satellites. Rescue is always at hand! But dangers remain. One of the greatest of these is an attitude of unquestioning acceptance and blind trust.

To find out and understand for oneself, to trust one's own judgment, may seem challenging. Central to this approach to therapy is the conviction that members of a group can themselves help one another through their insight and understanding. Therapists with this conviction do not set themselves up as knowing better than the rest. They may, through training, be blessed with a degree of understanding, but this is always in reserve, at the service of those they seek to help. Trusting people who do not have special training is at the heart of their work.

In this book we read how group analysis grew out of the 'one-to-one' practice of psychoanalysis and incorporates much psychoanalytic theory. When Foulkes broke with tradition and invited some of his patients to meet together in a group, conscious that from birth they had all been members of groups and were very largely formed by these, he believed they could only properly be understood in a group. He was in a group with them but did not lead the discussion, maintaining that he was there not to lead the group, nor to heal its members, but to trust them. In time they were able to shed much of their dependency and inhibiting assumptions about his authority. They could draw on their own insights to help one another in ways that went beyond the scope of one-to-one sessions in his consulting room.

The authors also describe the long and varied use of music in therapy in order to show how this, combined with group analysis, forms group music therapy.

As every culture uses music to express feelings and aspirations, so music has often been used to promote health. Islam, for instance, has a long tradition of music therapy. Treatises were written about the effects of music on the human soul and body; as early as the ninth century it was believed that melancholic diseases could be treated by listening to songs sung by beautiful voices. The Turkish scholar, Al-Farabi (870–950) was believed to make troubled people sleep when he played the lute. In the old hospital at Edirne in Turkey an orchestra played music to patients. Visitors there today can see displays that illustrate Islamic music therapy, and read that precise musical modes were prescribed for conditions such as heart disease, headaches and fevers, and for 'clearing the mind, increasing intelligence and refreshing memories'.

It is as hard to imagine a world without music as it is to picture a world without colour. The tunes and songs and rhythms that delight small children, our enjoyment of the work of great composers, music as an essential element in public ceremonies, and the satisfaction of joining together to make music in choirs, bands and orchestras, all enrich life. Daniel Barenboim (2001) observes that making music together teaches a valuable lesson about society: 'If you wish to learn how to live in a democratic society, then you would do well to play in an orchestra. For when you do so, you know when to lead and when to follow. You leave space for others and at the same time have no inhibitions about claiming a place for yourself.' So, in the same way, an analytic music therapy group where music is improvised sheds light on democracy: all contributions are distinctive, yet also simultaneous, and through them the group finds its collective voice.

In the last century music was used in psychiatric hospitals in England; celebrated professional musicians visited to perform before assembled patients. But that was passive listening. Then, soldiers traumatised in warfare were helped by making music together in groups as well as by discussion in group therapy. This had a powerful therapeutic effect, enabling them to confront deeply held and oppressive assumptions about the dangers they had faced. And today, improvising music together is found to help, amongst many others, children and adults with learning difficulties and patients with mental illness or dementia.

Music therapy has grown from these diverse roots. Now the insights of group analysis, together with active, improvised music making, give group music therapy increased potential to unlock deeply held psychological problems. In keeping with the spirit of this approach, students who are training to become music therapists will themselves be members of such groups and experience first-hand the possibilities they are preparing to offer to others.

Bill Lintott *is a member of the Institute of Group Analysis, London, and a founding member of Cambridge Group Work. He has conducted group analytic therapy groups in Cambridge and supervised those who conduct experiential groups for students in training to become music therapists.*

Preface

Eleanor Richards

Music therapy, like other psychological therapies, continues to be curious about the relationship between theoretical ideas and clinical practice. There is increasing research activity in both academic and clinical contexts, often related to work with particular patient groups, or to consideration of the place of the music within the therapeutic encounter.

In this book we examine some of the questions arising when we seek to investigate and establish theory in relation to group work. As much of the historical material in this book indicates, there is a long tradition of group work within music therapy in Britain. That is hardly surprising, perhaps; the social and relational nature of music itself readily implies the potential value of group music making in therapeutic settings. It is only relatively recently, however, that literature devoted to group music therapy has begun to appear. Some of that is concerned with offering suggestions for activities of a quite structured kind (Ramey 2011; Pinson 2013), some (e.g. Pavlicevic 2003) addresses similar issues but looks at them in the broader context of social theories about group life, and some (e.g. Grocke, Bloch and Castle 2009) is concerned with evaluating the outcomes and effectiveness of particular approaches. Discussion of group music therapy in analytic terms is also beginning to emerge (Davies and Richards 2002; Ahonen-Eerikainen 2011; Se Cho 2013). At the same time, analytic practitioners working in 'talking' therapies have found it useful to discuss events in language which draws very readily on the vocabulary of music. Foulkes, familiarly, talks of 'resonance' (and he preferred to think of the therapist as the 'conductor') and other authors have sought ways to articulate the musicality of the therapeutic encounter (Powell, A. 1983; Strich, S. 1983; Knoblauch, S. 2000; Stein, A. 1999). So something is going on; music therapy and group analysis are in conversation and group analysts, therefore, may find useful resources in the accounts here of group improvisation in music.

The preparation of this book has itself been, appropriately enough, a group endeavour. The three authors bring different perspectives, some with areas in common, some distinctive, and our hope is that the reader, as we have, will enjoy and pursue the creative possibilities inherent in the encounter between different minds, ideas, and experiences. In the same spirit, the book's material is presented in a range of ways which complement one another; there are accounts of theoretical and historical material, a conversation which brings some of that history to life through the experience of one clinician, some extended clinical material, and a series of shorter vignettes from contributors who are part of the wider group that has made this book possible.

The authors of this book come from different, though closely related, clinical backgrounds: Nick Barwick is a group analyst; Alison Davies and Eleanor Richards are music therapists who have also trained in analytic psychotherapy. As far as we are aware this is the first collaboration of its kind; our work together has been greatly enriched by time spent in discussion and by our experience of jointly running live workshops with groups of music therapists. Those events have included not only clinical and theoretical conversations, but also, vitally, group musical improvisations.

George Steiner (1997) points to some of the inherently contrasting elements in music which are, paradoxically, the source of its coherence:

> [Music's] forms in motion are at once more immediate and freer than those of language. By uses of inversion, of counterpoint, of polyphonic simultaneity, music can house contradictions, reversals of temporality, the dynamic coexistence within the same overall movement of wholly diverse, even mutually denying moods and pulses of feeling.
>
> Steiner (1997: 65–6)

That offers an image of any group that is alive. The meeting and mutual engagement of diverse people, and the musicality (in the broadest sense) of those encounters can bring something that is not simply 'greater than the sum of its parts', but enables each to flourish.

Acknowledgements

I would like to thank the Guildhall School of Music and Drama for its support, both with this project and with the development of my therapeutic interests over many years. As ever, I would also like to express special gratitude to my consultant, editor, confidante and wife, Carol, without whom, for me, much simply would not happen.

Nick Barwick

I am grateful to my supervisor, Bill Lintott, and to my colleague Sue Greenland, whose group analytic thinking and belief in groups have been inspirational.

Alison Davies

My thanks to Robert for his patience and encouragement, to many colleagues for enquiring and stimulating discussions, and to the Guildhall School of Music and Drama for its support for this undertaking.

Eleanor Richards

Part 1

Group music therapy
Historical perspectives

Chapter 1

Music therapy and the development of group work

Alison Davies

This chapter examines some of the significant developments in music therapy during the last half-century. These will be considered with a focus on the practice of music therapy in groups and on the ways in which analytic thinking has evolved within group music therapy.

There is no culture that is without music and for thousands of years music has been known to have been used in the context of healing in groups of people. Religious ceremonies and chanting come to mind, involving singing, drumming and other music as means of connecting to others and voicing shared emotion. The history of music therapy and its potential qualities for healing and restoring wellbeing have been substantially documented elsewhere; here I will focus on how the therapeutic use of music in groups has been introduced in healthcare and other settings and how the beginning of a more clinical and analytical approach to working therapeutically with groups in music has evolved.

Darnley-Smith and Patey (2003: 13), discussing the beginnings of working with music therapeutically, document the work of Dr Sydney Mitchell at Warlingham Park Hospital in the 1940s. This is of particular interest in the context of this book as it involved working with groups of people with music in a psychiatric setting. They also refer to an anonymous article 'Pioneers in Music Therapy', published in the bulletin of the British Society of Music Therapy in 1968.

One story exemplifies some of this work taking place in the late 1940s. An account is given of the work done by Sydney Mitchell and others who had conducted research and written 'many papers' on music therapy. At Warlingham Park Hospital, Mitchell had formed an orchestra of patients 'including string players, pianists and percussion instruments' where 'the primary object was the treatment rather than a high standard of performance'. He also analysed the effects of recorded music upon his patients, and whilst he found that 'classical music seemed to give a sense of security' he also found that 'the most effective means towards harmony of a group was folk songs and traditional music based upon the most deep-seated and cosmic relationship [which] strikes a psychological chord and brings people together' (2003: 13–14).

Of interest here is the idea that a certain sort of music is considered to bring harmony to a group and has the effect of bringing people together. This article also

4 Historical perspectives

describes work where 'live' music was used in a psychiatric setting by Drs Zanker and Glatt. Their conclusions were that

> patients' reactions to music can be of diagnostic value as they sometimes enabled the uncovering of unconscious attitudes. By helping to break down defences, fostering abreaction and bringing about emotional release music can be a therapeutic adjunct to other forms of therapy.
> BJMT (1968: 18–19) cited in Darnley-Smith and Patey (2003: 13)

In the late 1960s interest in the recognition of music as a therapeutic medium increased in the UK and Juliet Alvin established the first training course at the Guildhall School of Music and Drama in London in 1967. This developed out of an organisation called The Society for Music Therapy and Remedial Music, which was established in the late 1950s to gather together those interested in music therapy and to develop a professional practice. This later became the British Society for Music Therapy, a general organisation for all those interested in music therapy. Other professional training courses followed the one at the Guildhall School of Music and Drama, and the Association of Professional Music Therapists (APMT) was formed for those who had trained as music therapists. The first Research Fellowship was established in 1980 and music therapy, together with art therapy, was recognised by the NHS in 1982. Music therapy was later recognised professionally in 1988 by Social Services in England and Wales. Further and more detailed accounts of these milestones in the history of music therapy can be found in Darnley-Smith and Patey (2003: 16–22), but for the purposes of this chapter I will consider how an analytically informed approach developed and became one way of conceptualising the process and dynamics of group music therapy.

Mary Priestley was among the first to develop an analytic approach to music therapy. She worked in a psychiatric setting with patients with emotional and psychological disturbances. She and her colleagues pioneered their analytic approach to music therapy in the 1970s and 1980s at St. Bernard's Hospital in Middlesex. A century earlier, when this hospital was known as Hanwell Lunatic Asylum, its forward-thinking approaches to psychiatric care were already well established. St. Bernard's was known as early as 1955 for its linking of music therapy with psychotherapy; it was an ideal setting for Priestley to pioneer her analytical work. Priestley called her method Analytical Music Therapy (AMT) and described it as 'analytically-informed symbolic use of improvised music by the music therapist and client' (1994: 3).

Describing the early stages of Priestley's work, Darnley-Smith and Patey (2003) write:

> There was also a weekly music club, open to all on a voluntary basis. Patients heard about the sessions by word of mouth and came to find out what was happening, rather than by formal referral. The music club sessions contained

a mixture of spontaneous performances of singing and playing from the therapists and patients, as well as improvisation.

Darnley-Smith and Patey (2003: 25)

Priestley underwent her own psychoanalysis whilst she was undergoing her music therapy training. Her analytic approach developed out of her understanding of her own psychological processes. She believed that having personal analysis was important if the therapist was to have insight into her patient's inner world. On the whole, up until then, music therapists practised without necessarily thinking actively about the complexities of the psyche. During the 1980s, however, it became increasingly common for students to have their own therapy. In due course it became a mandatory requirement for training.

Mary Priestley wrote:

> As I was in analysis with Dr Wooster at the time [of music therapy training] I was being made aware of subtler, more problematic, and often more conflicting workings of the psyche, with conscious and unconscious moving in different directions, sapping the vital energy and causing confusion in the thinking and subsequent behaviour.
>
> Priestley (1994: 129)

She goes on to describe some of the Kleinian and Freudian concepts as well as the language of dreams that influenced her analytical thinking. During her training she was also greatly influenced by Alfred Nieman, a composer and teacher of improvisation on the music therapy training at the Guildhall School of Music and Drama.

She quotes Nieman, who during her training said:

> Music faces us with the realisation that there are two worlds: the inner and the outer. The inner is often incommunicable, a spiritual world which is difficult to enter from the outer world where we normally speak to one another. Music is a bridge for us by which we can reach this inner world. That is why free improvisation is so vital for music therapy. You are privileged people to be able to communicate with this deepest part of human beings.
>
> Priestley (1994: 31)

Priestley found this a very significant statement in the light of her future work as a music therapist. Like Nieman, she focused on music's capacity for wordless articulation of feeling and its potential for bringing unconscious material into awareness. Here she describes her own quasi-therapeutic group with colleagues and how it was informed by her understanding of psychoanalysis.

> Analytical Music Therapy (AMT) was developed while I was working as a music therapist with three colleagues in a large psychiatric hospital and while

having my own Kleinian psychoanalysis ... We met in the basement flat weekly for ninety-six sessions trying out different experimental techniques using improvised music, usually on instruments but sometimes including vocal expression. We usually used a focus in the form of a title with which the mind could direct the emotions ... Although most of the techniques were developed out of our desire to help our patients with their problems, some were the clarification of our own problems following up work that had been done in our own analysis. Occasionally something would come from a workshop one of us had attended, thus there were some techniques which nod to Gestalt Therapy and Psycho-synthesis. We gave each other feedback on the results of the experimental techniques and I took careful notes in my diary ...

Priestley (1994: 1–2)

Mary Priestley called this way of working 'Intertherap' and her main focus was to use music as a creative way of accessing and exploring aspects of emotional life that may be obscured, rather than clarified, by language. This experience helped her and students in training to develop ways of working analytically. She said that to practise in this way the music therapist needs to know how to translate what is explored verbally and felt emotionally into musical expression. She emphasised the difference between how we relate in words and how we relate in music. She stated that music, or 'sound expression' as she called it, allows a greater closeness and openness to feelings in the therapeutic relationship.

Music therapists have subsequently drawn upon many of these aspects of Priestley's work when working analytically. Thinking with her clients about their improvised music was often in very symbolic terms. She believed that this acted as a creative tool through which to 'explore the client's inner life so as to provide the way forward for growth and greater self knowledge' and she speaks of

the joy of being able to share non-verbally with the therapist a life-enhancing inner and outer happening, the experience of harmonious and beautiful rhythms, interactions, or the reassurance of being able to survive a wildly chaotic or dissonant musical interaction and end in peace and friendship.

Priestley (1994: 3–4)

Attending to the atmosphere and sense of the relationship in therapy Priestley goes on to say that sometimes the experience encountered together with patients was that of just 'sitting together in chosen silence, feeling the harmonious non-necessity of words until the time feels right to speak' (1994: 5). Priestley is describing a 'being together' with neither words nor music where the atmosphere containing a kind of 'music' in itself is of value in the growing relationship. What is being communicated is a different, wordless understanding or knowingness between the therapist and patient. This other place of relatedness that she describes, waiting in silence until the moment when the time feels appropriate to speak, seems to have come from her own experience in analysis. This is interesting when thinking about times in groups when no words are said or music played and where there may be many different versions of the same silence going on at the same time for group members.

Priestley's intention was that the therapeutic relationship, articulated through shared improvisational music, would lead to a better way of relating outside therapy. She was helping the client's growing ability, through the music, to trust an intimacy and closeness which had the potential to lead to a more authentic way of relating to others. In what she describes as 'guided expression of the music' (1994: 7) she noticed that the patient's resistance to denied or split-off feelings and emotions could be reduced because the threshold of consciousness was lowered. She felt that emotions expressed symbolically through sound or movement might allow the experience to be less painful and that these emotions could lead to 'vivid memories and inner images' (1994: 7). Music, she felt, enabled repressed material to surface, thus allowing it to be worked through to consciousness. She pointed to the idea that an impulse released in music could be understood or expressed in various ways. It 'can either be accepted or partly accepted, or it can be sublimated, used in a constructive and creative way and harmless way or it can be consciously condemned' (1994: 7).

Another interesting approach described by Priestley, this time linked to negative transference, relates to how aggression might be held in the music:

> through the musical expression aggressive and auto-aggressive tendencies can be externalised in sound without the therapist succumbing to the assault. This relieves the patient of the guilt of having to create verbal channels of hate and destructiveness which might be better left unverbalised
>
> Priestley (1994: 7–8)

She describes this as positive use of anger rather than its negative assertion. It is as if the instruments take the force of the transference.

Central to Priestley's way of working was the training of students by giving them the experience of their own Intertherap as part of their personal development as music therapists. Students would improvise music together taking turns in being the patient and then the therapist. This way of working in music therapy did not really take root in the UK in the way that it did in Germany, where it was developed by Johannes Eschen, one of the first to be trained in Intertherap by Mary Priestley.

Paul Nordoff, an American pianist and composer, and Clive Robbins, a teacher, were also pioneers in music therapy practice in the UK, taking a rather different approach. Their musical partnership originated in collaborative work, primarily with children with special needs. Although their work in groups focused on a more social and educative approach, aspects of the ways they were working are important to consider in relation to this book. They had no single method that they regarded as gospel; instead they emphasised the necessity to find and meet the needs of the child in the music of each individual.

They wrote: 'all the techniques we give you must be modified, adapted, even ignored, depending on the children you work with. Otherwise music therapy becomes a prescription and a dogma and an uncreative activity' (quoted in Aigen 1996: 32).

Working together, they helped the child with learning difficulties to participate musically. Paul Nordoff played improvised music on the piano, whilst Clive Robbins helped to facilitate the child's musical interactions. The music (which included the singing voice) mirrored, responded to, and amplified the sound contributions of the child.

Nordoff, interviewed for BBC TV in 1976, said:

> We meet the tempo in whatever the child is doing, the tempo of his walking, his head banging, his pacing up and down, his rocking. We take the sounds he might make, whether it is screaming or screaming-crying, and we give this back to him in music so that he has a new experience of what he does habitually. And then, gradually, the goals we have to work for emerge as the child shows us. 'Here I am, this is me, I can only do this.'
>
> Nordoff (1976) quoted in Darnley-Smith and Patey (2003: 31)

Nordoff and Robbins often composed music in the form of songs that reflected the natural rhythms of the child's speech. This enabled the child to learn the songs and their melodies easily. The child's movement was also mirrored in the music. Attention was paid to the harmonies and rhythms that supported the music in both song and music for movement. Thoughtful use of dissonance to reflect mood were also important and they considered that this enabled the child to move with determination as well as helping them to learn the words for songs and guiding them through the musical games.

They wrote:

> Throughout the game, through the dynamic mood of the music, [the children] would awaken to the situation in which they found themselves. The dissonances not only enabled them to march and move with more vigour, but helped them to learn and remember the words and melodies.
>
> Nordoff and Robbins (1973: 22)

Nordoff and Robbins describe the early musical groups they convened at Sunfield House in Worcestershire, in which musical games accompanied the enactment of stories. A story such as 'Pif-Paf-Poltrie' (from a Brothers Grimm fairy tale) or 'The Three Bears' would evolve into a structured musical experience with these children. Active participation included singing, dancing, action dialogue, marching and moving together as the story unfolded through music and movement. This helped the children to enter together into a rich and intense experience of both the story and each other through experiencing the music together. Each child then had the possibility of experiencing an increased awareness and sense of themselves with others in a social setting. The aim was to let the music stimulate the emotional development of the child. In terms of a group, having access to the 'music child' in one another, to use their term, could ameliorate the sense of isolation for group members and help them to communicate in a social and group environment.

I have emphasised the value of the social belonging and connectivity of these musical activities developed by Nordoff and Robbins. In the chapter of this book discussing early development (Chapter 8) there is further discussion of the importance of singing and rhythmical sounds in the emotional stimulation and development of children's speech and of how musical interactions of this kind can be avenues of connection for those with communication difficulties as well as helping to create a social setting of inclusion.

Elaine Streeter, a music therapist and music therapy trainer, in her foreword to the *Journal of British Music Therapy* (1987) describes the use of music therapy in two different ways, reflecting alternative approaches.

Firstly, she describes the 'use of music in order to stimulate the patient's interest in an activity which is, in itself, therapeutic for him' (1987: 3). The music in this instance would be chosen by the therapist to help him, for example, make 'a movement or produce a sound which the therapist has previously determined as beneficial for him' (1987: 3). In a group context this could take the form of a structured greeting song with clients who find difficulty in recognising and connecting to others in the group. The music of the song might draw out and stimulate the musicality within the adult or the child and through the skill of the therapist the client could be helped to connect and reach out to others in the group.

Secondly, Streeter describes the ability of the music therapist to encourage the patients to express themselves creatively in the music. Through musical improvisation with the therapist, the creativity of the patient has the potential to be unlocked. The therapeutic value here could be twofold. Firstly, the unfolding of musical creativity could bypass the disability of the client; secondly, it could bring the patient and the therapist into connection and communication with each other, thus developing and deepening a therapeutic relationship. Again, in reference to improvisation in a group setting, being in a music therapy group fosters a sense of being together through the contribution of each person's sound or, in some cases, silence. This can go far in helping to ameliorate a sense of aloneness and isolation. Streeter describes a further use of music that is 'based on the idea that certain types of music can stimulate particular states of mind, emotions or images . . . the therapist uses a form of creative intuition that reflects the feelings of the client at the time' (1987: 3–4). Translated into group terms, this could take the form of the music therapist (or possibly the patients themselves) suggesting that the group play music that reflects the perceived feeling amongst them in the room. It is interesting to note here that a group improvising without preliminary discussion will often naturally play music that expresses the dynamics that are at play at that particular moment, whether it be togetherness and uniformity or resistance and conflict.

David John, in his paper 'Towards Music Psychotherapy' (1992), begins to explore an area of working in music therapy that is related to a psychoanalytic approach. He views the music as an attempt to create a link, or 'build a bridge' as he puts it, between unconscious and conscious processes. He pays debt to others such as Heal (1989; 1992), Priestley (1975), and Towse (1991), who had also looked in the direction of psychoanalysis to conceptualise aspects of their work. John developed various psychoanalytic concepts in relation to music; here he outlines the psychological phenomena that constitute a primarily Freudian view – including defence mechanisms, conscious and unconscious processes, instinctual drives, and transference/counter transference – and shows how he views music in light of these theories. His proposal is that the music can be viewed in several ways:

- As a product of an organizing and communicative component of the mental apparatus;
- As a substitute for an instinctual representation;
- As an object onto which can be projected subjective experience (fantasies and feeling);
- As a symbolic representation of states of mental conflict;
- As a symbolic representation of the working of the mental apparatus;
- As a benign external stimulus.

John (1992)

Music, he suggests, can be a way of relieving the 'tyranny of the inhibitory factors operating in the mind' and can provide a 'relief from narcissistic withdrawal and isolation, through offering a means of organising a relation with an external object (the therapist)' (1992: 12).

John Woodcock, who was at the time practising as a music therapist at Warley Hospital in Essex, published a paper in the *Journal of British Music Therapy* (1987) entitled 'Towards Group Analytic Music Therapy'. He describes his work with adult patients who did not have any significant psychotic element in their pathology and who had sufficient sense of self to be able to reflect on the process of the group. Woodcock was one of the first music therapists to use and to write about a group analytically informed approach to work with groups; he derived his thinking about music therapy groups from the group analytic theories and techniques primarily of S.H. Foulkes. He considered Foulkes' use of an unstructured group where the group as a whole is held in mind and where the therapist follows the lead of the group and, in the service of the group, looks on his role of conductor as a catalytic agent (S.H. Foulkes 1964: 57). Woodcock also draws on the theory of Wilfred Bion's three basic assumptions of dependency, flight/fight and pairing in a group, which Bion discusses extensively in his book *Experiences in Groups* (Bion 1961). All these group analytic techniques and ways of working were thought about in relation to dynamics that could be observed in both the talking and the musical improvisation. Woodcock tackles the often-controversial area of talking versus the playing of music in music therapy, which at that time (the mid-1980s) was much debated.

In a paper in the *British Journal of Psychotherapy* (1991) Esme Towse takes up the analytic theory of transference in relation to the music in a music therapy group. Quoting Sandler et al. (1973), she understands transference to be

> a specific illusion which develops in regard to the other person, which, unbeknown to the subject, represents in some of its features, a repetition of a relationship towards an important figure in the person's past . . . it should be emphasised that this is felt by the subject, not as a repetition of the past, but as strictly appropriate to the present and to the particular person involved.
>
> cited in Towse (1991)

Towse looks at how the transference might play out in the music of the group. In thinking about the resolution of transference issues she says that group members can learn and become aware of the reactions of themselves and others in both the words and the music. She argues that the value of the music is the possibility of understanding, through the music, the effect on others of one's playing before moving on and bringing these thoughts into words. She observes that this seems to be because of the less threatening nature of the music. Yet, paradoxically, she also says that a music therapy group can be more provocative than a verbal therapy group because it may be easier to think how one's music might affect others, as it is more direct in the here and now.

Finally, this chapter cannot be concluded without mention of the work of Helen Odell-Miller, interviewed elsewhere in this book, who in the 1980s set up a music therapy service in a psychiatric setting where there was a history of social therapy organised along therapeutic community lines. Although commitment to a therapeutic community model in psychiatry has been very much eroded in recent decades, the 1980s and 1990s saw many music therapists drawing on psychoanalytically informed theory in particular with their work in music therapy groups.

Odell-Miller (2001) writes about how her music therapy group work 'reflects both a musically and a psychoanalytically informed way of working' (2001: 138). She describes how the active musical improvisations of group members together can provide both an intense and emotionally shared experience and an insight for the therapist into a greater understanding of the group as a whole as well as its individual members. She draws attention to a unique aspect of group music making, which is that all members of the group have the possibility to play and so 'talk' (as it were) at once. Thus the whole feeling of the group can be observed through the improvised music that is produced. She refers to the ongoing dialogue amongst music therapists as to the balance between the music and verbal contributions in groups, and looks at the development of interpersonal and intrapersonal relationships that unfold during the group process.

Chapter 2

The development of group work in music therapy in the UK

Helen Odell-Miller in conversation with Eleanor Richards

Helen Odell-Miller is Professor of Music Therapy at Anglia Ruskin University, Cambridge, and has practised music therapy since 1976. She currently works as a researcher, trainer and therapist. She has published and lectured widely and is a strong advocate of music therapy in mental health services. She pioneered music therapy services in Cambridge, with a focus on group work at Fulbourn Hospital with adults with mental health problems, within an approach grounded in therapeutic communities. She was an instigator of the amalgamation of arts therapies services nationally and locally; that stemmed from her experience of working with other arts therapists and seeing how groups functioned using arts media to work towards therapeutic change.

I'm interested in your earliest experience in music therapy in relation to groups. How was group work addressed during your training at the Guildhall?
I don't remember any theoretical training, in terms of group analytic theory or even social theory, about groups; Juliet Alvin [then head of the training] was very keen on looking at group interactions, but not really in psychodynamic terms. We didn't have a group in the way that an experiential training group might be run now; we had weekly group improvisation training with Alfred Nieman. I think that was the only place – with my fellow students – that I really tried working in groups as part of my training process.

What did you understand Juliet Alvin to mean by 'interaction'?
She was very much concerned with cause and effect, so she would bring her cello, for example, into the student group, and then get us to try things out, but it was more in terms of exercises than reflection on the group process: 'I play this and, oh look, your eyes lit up there, and then you followed my beat, or you didn't follow my beat.' We talked about casework, in more of a behaviour-oriented way than happens on UK trainings now, but very musically based. The weekly group with Alfred Nieman was more like a free improvisation agenda-less group. A lot of dynamics were unfolding, of course, but they were never discussed except in terms of giving feedback to individual students. He would ask the group to improvise freely, but within particular idioms: atonally, for instance.

Was that particularly directed towards group work?
It was with us as a group, but there was no reflection about what might be happening between us psychologically. But he might say, 'Helen, you just didn't listen to that person over there' or 'Ian, you didn't follow her beat' or 'Helen, it's your turn. Here's a theme or a topic, and we'll see what the group does with it, but you're the leader.' But he would analyse it in musical terms. On reflection, I remember that I found it quite hard, because I'm quite sensitive musically, but also I was aware that there was other stuff going on. Sometimes someone would just get hold of a beat and be enraged and stamp across somebody else's music. But there was no reflection on that in psychological terms; they might just have said something like 'Well, that was a bit of a muddle and none of you were listening to each other.'

Was that at a stage in the development of music therapy training when people were not in their own personal therapy?
They may have been for their own reasons, but there was no requirement to be in individual therapy, and no ongoing process looked at in the group. I can remember quite a lot of very powerful feelings being evoked within me and probably within all of us, but they were never spoken about.

So did those musical experiences in groups with Alfred Nieman get transferred into teaching about the possibilities of clinical practice, when you started to work with patients?
Not in terms of how to manage a group, or how to think about working in a group.

So how were you prepared for placements in terms of group work?
Sometimes we tried things out with each other, more with Maggie Pickett [another member of GSMD staff] than with Juliet Alvin. We were prepared in this sort of master class way, where we'd all be in a group, and then Maggie would say something like 'Today we're going to look at action songs'. So you might imagine you were running a group with people with learning disabilities and you wanted them to know more about their body parts; it was quite concrete. And then we would work together, and perhaps go off to compose something and then come back and try it with the group. And that's the only thing I can remember about any group training. But there was no process thought about, and it was quite spasmodic.

What are your memories of your early clinical group work when you were training?
My first experience of a group was at St Charles psychiatric hospital with Juliet Alvin, and there were no groups similar to the types of groups I've experienced since then, because there was a change each week as to where she'd work, who she'd work with, and what she'd do. I also spent some with Maggie Pickett at the Charing Cross service, where she ran an acute psychiatric group;

it was a very large, chaotic group on an acute ward, where everyone seemed to be sitting at different levels all over the ward and in the middle of the sitting area. And if I think about that now, I would have called it a community-oriented music therapy group, in that it was a group using music in the middle of the environment, and probably was a reflection of what was going on in that environment. But unless I just wasn't picking up on this, it didn't seem to be considered in depth; there was more interest in cause and effect, in what the therapist did and how that affected the group. And there was quite a lot of performing going on by the therapist. So I would say now that I could perhaps put a theoretical model on that, but it wasn't really thought about.

What did you learn from doing that group?
I think all the way through my training I learnt a lot about myself and about working in groups; it made me seek ways of thinking, I suppose, about models of how the work could be done. So in this first placement, there was a psychiatric unit, but we didn't go there much; we went to the acute wards where people were recovering from surgery. I remember going into a ward of men who'd had amputations, and we would go to each person's space. Juliet would have her cello. It was very chaotic. And sometimes she would say 'Well, would any men like to gather round?' and then she'd just improvise. She'd sing, or she'd work with a song that someone brought. It could happen anywhere in the ward. So there wasn't the idea that you would set aside a space, within which a group would have an experience that you might reflect on. It was more a sort of studio group, so anything could happen. It was good training, because it taught me how to deal with anything, and any emotional situation. She would throw you in the deep end and start to do music with people, and then afterwards tell you whether you'd got the pace or the rhythm or the harmonic progressions right. (This was long ago!) So I think it was very good for learning to think on my feet. It meant that I was very relaxed when I went to the Ida Darwin [a large learning disability hospital near Cambridge] and was actually doing quite big groups there in music and movement with physiotherapists. But it made me realise I wanted to have things like a beginning and an ending time, and more thought about the process.

And in those settings, where you were as a student, did you encounter other clinicians who thought analytically working with groups?
I think when I went to Charing Cross there were people there, but I didn't meet them. My main placements were St Charles (the training was only a year long), then in a school for people with autism, and then at the Ida Darwin, where I did almost entirely group work, in fact. They had advertised a full time post, and for some reason nobody applied and so Tony Wigram relinquished a day at another job he was doing, and worked there temporarily, to keep it open. And I went there on placement. Later a post was advertised and I was appointed, but it was on placement that I learnt a lot about working in groups, but again not

from a psychoanalytic perspective. Tony Wigram had a natural gift for picking up on the mood and atmosphere of the group. So we ran small and large groups and there was structure. So that's really where I learned about having a beginning and middle and end, and thinking about the process. But again, it was on the level of working with the way that people used music, but working with their feelings in the moment.

So what were your clinical objectives with that learning disabled population?
Tony Wigram was very organised about that, so each patient would have an individual aim that might be to do with motivation, or awareness of other people, or interaction. I think I probably brought the idea of group aims in later. Although it was implicit as to why people were in a group, group events were not much discussed, other than that we would sit down afterwards and say 'Well, that was quite hard to manage', or 'Wasn't it difficult when X was singing at the top of his voice?', and we would wonder whether we had managed that well or not. So it was all the stuff of groups, but without any sort of any psychological theory.

It sounds, particularly knowing what we do of Tony Wigram, as though it was very musically oriented.
Yes. I think I was always thinking about the psychological aspects, but I didn't have particular models until I met Mary Priestley during my training. I went to see her, to talk to her more about 'intertherap' and her method, and I read her book while I was at the Ida Darwin. I remember that this way of wondering about what's going on internally for people, and how that might be reflected in the music, started to interest me.

So it was a catalyst coming across her and her work?
Yes. Another catalyst was encounters with some occupational therapy colleagues I worked with when I started the job there. Then I really began to learn, as I was running groups myself. I worked sometimes with the physiotherapists, sometimes on my own or with nursing staff. I ran some quite chaotic groups on wards, to try and engage people who were extremely disabled and lying on the floor, sometimes not fully clothed, sometimes incontinent. Perhaps I was learning from the way that Alfred Nieman worked; I was comfortable with just using music to reflect what was going on, in a very free way.

It's interesting that in that approach is something that group analytic thinking might also recognise: perhaps there isn't anybody who's inherently unsuitable for a group.
I learnt later about that. I really wanted to go and work at Fulbourn Hospital. Some OT colleagues there were interested in learning about group work through going on training weekends, usually with other arts therapists, or through things like psychodrama training groups, working with Veronica Sherbourne, who did

some of the early music and movement therapy work, and Sue Jennings. I became involved in that, all the time starting to think about ways that this group work might translate into music therapy. Through that a group of us formed something called Scope, which changed later to a specific group for arts therapists, but at that point was open to OTs and arts therapists and others who were interested in group processes. I suppose it developed from the sixties encounter group movement, and probably some of the people who came to those weekends worked at Fulbourn Hospital in the psychiatric service, and had worked with people like David Clark, who was running a lot of groups there. He had worked with Maxwell Jones, the initiator of therapeutic communities.

Did you go to those weekends just to enhance your music therapy practice, or were you also going for yourself?
I was going for my own process. I hadn't had any personal therapy at this point.

Was that part of what alerted you to the possibility of working at Fulbourn?
I wanted to experiment in running music therapy groups with people who weren't so learning disabled. I was wondering whether if I worked with people who weren't so impaired, these processes might be able to happen through music therapy. So I did two things. I enrolled for Cambridge Group Work, where I was in a group led by a pair of co-therapists, Ronald Spiers and Inge Hudson, and that was a turning point for me, because it was agenda-less and unstructured. So that was the nearest I'd been to having my own therapy, I suppose. And the group work was supported by theoretical seminars. It was validated by the IGA.

That sounds like an exciting time.
Yes. It was brilliant. I was having my own experience, but all the time I was thinking 'How does this relate to music?' and noticing points when I thought music could come into it – or not. There was another woman in the group who was a play therapist, and she was (unlike me, actually) very frustrated by the lack of actually doing stuff. But I do remember thinking 'If this group suddenly played, I wonder what it would sound like?' At the same time, the Scope group that we formed met on Saturdays and we did work with each other. I mentioned to Sue Beecraft (an OT) that I would really like to try out music therapy in psychiatry and try to set up a post at Fulbourn; she suggested that first I got some experience. So we ran a group together for about nine months with a group of people who were homeless and who also had mental health problems, and were in and out of Fulbourn.

Rather like an acute group?
Yes. And through that, I began to develop a model in my mind of group music therapy.

It's striking that you were in the group at Cambridge Group Work, and wondering what the group might sound like if they moved out of the words into the music. It's a very interesting turnaround, isn't it?
Absolutely. And vice versa too. I got to value thinking and reflecting and talking; sometimes in very articulate groups it was easy for the music to get a bit lost, especially the more I had group analytic supervision and did more group analytic training. But I've always thought that the balance is very important in group music therapy. So Sue and I did that work and then wrote it up. David Clark invited us to come and do a presentation at Fulbourn; we had permission to play some of the musical examples, and we spoke about it to a large gathering of nursing staff, psychologists and psychiatrists. And on the strength of that, they decided to convert a mixture of an entertainment post and a tailor's post into a music therapy post. It was advertised and I was appointed. I spent three months going around, just inducting myself within all the different units and running staff groups with music, in order to see whether music therapy would be suitable in that unit. And then, on the strength of that, my work at Fulbourn started; they had art therapy then but not music therapy. But everything was centred around groups, because David Clark had learnt a lot from Maxwell Jones, and worked in other therapeutic communities. Actually there was so much emphasis on the group that sometimes it took a long time for decisions to be made.

Really?
The group would sit and think about things for a long time; the meetings were often run through using art, or the art therapists would work in a meeting at the same time as the group was trying to deal with its business.

It sounds a wonderfully spacious time.
There was no pressure about seeing hundreds of patients. There was an emphasis on the staff being looked after, so every unit had a staff support group; an arts therapist sometimes ran that. That seemed like bread and butter for the staff; there was very little questioning about getting together and doing it, in fact people were pleased to. And there was sometimes conflict in what was called the parliament meeting, which was the weekly meeting between all staff who worked in the rehabilitation unit; David Clark ran it like a large group. So we were doing business but there was no agenda, and people would say what was on their minds, and the business would emerge. And when there was disagreement about different attitudes and ways of doing things; at least a few times I remember them saying 'Why don't we look at this through an art form?' By then there was a drama therapist too, and he might do something in order to look at the process. I ran quite a few music therapy groups with the staff, on a one-off basis, to look at a particular dynamic. It seemed like second nature. Staff would come in and think 'I really want to get to grips with this'. There was conflict and debate and people would fall out, but it was all part of the process, and there was time. Although each unit had a staff support group, there was also an emphasis on the community. So in

each section, like the elderly service, which had lots of different wards and units, or particularly in the rehab unit, which David Clark ran, everyone would gather, probably once a week, in meetings which were rather like large groups.

It's very interesting that there were nursing staff actively convinced of the value of using the arts in their own process. That's remarkable, isn't it? How did that analytic thinking, which you took in through things like Cambridge Group Work and the staff groups at Fulbourn, begin to inform your clinical practice with patients?
A major way was through supervision. An arts therapies casework supervision group was set up, and that's really where I started to gain a proper understanding of analytic thinking. The first supervisor was Graham Davis; he worked analytically, but he was also very sensitive to other dimensions. He'd thought a lot about group analytic practice, and how that theory could inform working without the spoken word. But he was very challenging. So he would question the idea (particularly in individual work, so this might not be so relevant), of 'acting'; he would consider the possibility of acting out with clients, if you're involved in, say, improvising together at the piano. Somebody presented a case each week, and then we would reflect on it together. But he would not only think psychoanalytically about the work using spoken language and words; he would also sometimes get up and use his body – a psychodynamic body orientation – to get into things more deeply. Neville Symington talks about the importance in analytic work of the analyst actually being *in* the relationship, not just being there *for* somebody. And I think I learnt about that possibility through a lot of the teaching from Graham in the supervision group; he would take musical examples, and he would seem to have to get into it, by getting up and using a cushion, or putting it into movement, and almost enacting it or getting into some form of embodiment, and then come back and comment psychodynamically and musically about what was going on. It was very interesting. And we actually did a project where we started to think about how the supervision group was informing our thinking and informing the development of some of the models that some of us were then going away and developing on the wards, in group and individual work; we started to video the supervision group, to see what the components were, and what was happening that was informing our work. So there was a research dimension that came in, that again arose from the clinical experience, where some of us thought it would be interesting to look at this a bit more systematically, and so we did some work with that; there was a culture of learning.

Was this ground breaking, or were there other places where the same sorts of developments were unfolding?
I think in terms of the arts therapies, this was quite ground breaking, although I think there were arts therapists in comparable places, like the Cassel and the Henderson.

And music therapy in particular?
I joined the Association of Therapeutic Communities. When I went to Fulbourn I worked on Street Ward, where the whole of the patients' week was oriented towards thinking about themselves in relation to the community. There was a community meeting every morning, where all the staff and patients sat together and reflected on what had been going on overnight and the previous day and in the moment. The idea was that the way that people were relating in the community was thought about in every way, in every setting. Through the ATC I did encounter other arts therapists, but not many music therapists. And so within the APMT we set up the Psychiatric Interest Group, which was helpful in establishing some new posts. There was a group of us who started to meet regularly and think about the interface between the arts therapies and psychoanalytic theory.

John Woodcock wrote a paper about group analytic music therapy for the first ever edition of the British Journal of Music Therapy. Did that come out of those discussions?
Some of his thinking did, I think. In addition, most of us who were engaged in that work were having our own analysis. I didn't do formal training, because I wanted to be a music therapist, interestingly, although I thought about it. David John joined our service in the mid-eighties, and he brought more analytic thinking; a lot of us did a kind of training where we would take on a patient and be supervised in the psychotherapy department. So that was not just with Graham Davis, but with John Sklar and Colin James and other analysts.

And they were doing group work?
Yes. Then Colin James set up much more intensive weekends at Fulbourn, using the IGA model of being in a small group and then a large group. One of my first experiences was being in a group with Meg Sharpe as the group analyst; she must be one of the earliest members of the IGA, and interestingly is also a musician. I think she published a paper about music and analysis, but it wasn't about music therapy. So that was after the therapeutic community phase. Then came a more, I suppose, psychoanalytic phase; a more individualistic model as well came in after one of the White Papers, where there was a criticism of psychiatric services in that they didn't focus enough on people's individual needs, and that's where care plans started to develop. And there was something of a move away from the emphasis on group process at that point, and a bit of a decline in therapeutic communities. But at the same time Colin James brought in this group analytic training, which had a huge momentum, and revived a different and much more analytic way of thinking about groups.

Do you have a sense of how that more analytic thinking about groups got disseminated through our profession? What was the place of the APMT, for instance, in that, or what were related developments in MT trainings?
There was a big turning point, where some of us who'd started to do analytic work ourselves had had some therapy, and also those who had done some experiential

work in groups wanted to experiment more with music therapy in that way. A key institution there was Roehampton Institute, where Elaine Streeter and Pamela Steele were running the training. Elaine Streeter and I – I don't know which year this was, but it was some time in the late eighties – were both involved in the APMT and we decided to take some of this group experiential thinking into the organisation. So on the Fulbourn model of doing your work as a therapist, but at the same time reflecting on it as you go along, in groups, we decided to run an experiential residential weekend in Cambridge. It took a similar form to one of the IGA models: a combination of small and large group formats.

But working with music . . .
. . . but working with music. And we employed Vega Roberts to be a sort of group analytic supervisor to the people running the groups. I didn't run one; I wanted to be in one. There were three or four groups, and we worked in these small groups intensively. The one I was in was run as an analytic group really, but with music.

And dialogue?
Yes. There was some dialogue, quite a bit of it, but then a move into improvisation and then a move back into words. I think that event was a big turning point.

So what made it a turning point? Was it that people came who hadn't hitherto met that way of thinking?
Yes. It was also a meeting of minds between people who had started to look at the interface between music therapy and psychoanalytic thinking. I think one of the major questions was: what can happen if the therapist doesn't play? I think there was an agreement over that weekend that the therapist didn't play. So they took what I think they thought was a stance that an analyst might take, through listening and interpretation, but they decided not to play music with their groups. And I think that's very interesting; I can see that that was probably an important moment.

What did you make of that personally? Did you welcome it?
I thought it was very helpful at one level, because it threw the group into their own process. But the other thing I reflected on, probably not necessarily then or in the moment, was the idea that if the music therapist decides as a rule that they will not play, then they are not using their musical understanding and skill to facilitate or help the process develop, or indeed give some different musical meaning to the musical process. So although something might be gained, something also might be missing, because that would be a bit like the analyst never speaking or never using their mind, or voicing their feelings.

That brings to my mind the familiar idea that everybody in the group is changed by the experience, including the therapist, and I think that's inevitable; if one's in a group in any capacity one is changed. But it's an interesting model, that the therapist doesn't articulate musically her part in that process.

It was very powerful. I think some people in the group were quite angry about it. There were some more traditionally trained music therapists who found it difficult to understand. But on the other hand I suppose one could say that we were the group as well, and we were all musicians and music therapists, and we were playing together, and that what the therapist did was listen intensely and comment on what she heard happening, not in very personal terms, but more about the music; because that was her style in those days, to consider how people were listening and how they seemed to be making music. So she was using her musical understanding in a way that someone who isn't a musician might not have been able to do, including talking about modulation and affect. So it's assumed in my model that the work is about trying to help people manage and think about the meaning of events, particularly in terms of their feelings. I suppose the thing that might have been missing there [at the conference] is the way that a music therapist in a group could reflect musically the affect of the group, or play something that's implied or nearly there, but the group haven't really articulated.

Do you think that the experience of that conference fed back into what happened on training courses, in terms of the curriculum and ways of thinking about preparing people to be clinicians?
Absolutely. That sort of experience is now the bread and butter of student training on many courses in the UK; at least once a week for quite an intensive period, students are having a similar experience, in a music therapy group, often run by somebody who is doubly trained, who's got experience in using that dimension of helping the group feel what it's like to work through musical interaction not only for themselves, but to understand something about the group and the group process. I remember it changing the whole way I worked with groups in the clinical setting, in the sense that I did less. I didn't *not* play – particularly in acute settings, I would still play, but I would also leave a lot more to the group to work out for themselves. And that's what that experience did for me. I am not sure, but I think we might have been the first training course to include a music therapy group experience every week in an intensive way when we set up the training course at Anglia.

Well, there was a group like that when I trained at Roehampton in the 1990s. But it was run by someone who was also a member of staff, so that boundary wasn't there at that stage. But on the other hand we were all in therapy, so we each had a separate space too.
When we set the training course up at Anglia, we recommended everyone was in therapy, and most people were, but it wasn't required. But within that we definitely set up very intensive experiential groups. One was run by Elaine Streeter and one by David John for the first few years. And then you came, and Alison Davies. We thought that was a crucial learning experience. And then other trainings took it on board, but I think it did probably originate from Roehampton in the beginning.

Right from the beginning as well, we used an experiential music therapy group, to interview trainees, and that was something that we introduced. Amelia Oldfield designed the course with me, and I think certainly she would have been very keen that people were assessed musically. But maybe the sort of more group dynamic experience on the interview day came from my background of the group culture at Fulbourn. For years we had been involving people in a group if they came for an interview there. In 1985 I went on a Churchill Fellowship and we needed to employ a locum; we put the candidates into a music therapy improvisation setting, and said 'It's about your motivation and reasons for coming to apply for this job'. We also encouraged candidates to work through each art form. Music therapy seemed to lend itself to immediate here-and-now models of group work that worked very well in that situation. In fact we felt that we couldn't really decide if people were appropriate for the job unless we'd seen them in that type of setting.

And you translated that into the student selection process?
Yes, then that influenced the training, but none of this is my thinking alone. It's hard to trace all the influences.

Do you have a sense now – and it may be reflected in what we do at Anglia anyway – about how we might best prepare students to work clinically with groups, in terms of both theoretical ideas and experiential work?
I'll try and be succinct but this is quite important. When you're very experienced you might be able to work more on your own. When Amelia Oldfield and I set the training up, we'd both worked for many years, and we used that experience to design a training course, but a mistake we made was not to focus enough on how the students could help each other. So in the early years we had a few case discussion groups and the students had their experiential group, but there wasn't so much focus on the group process as part of students' learning process in lectures and workshops. It was happening in a way, but we didn't emphasise it enough. So we realised that some students felt quite isolated, because they were receiving individual clinical supervision. A few years in we realised that that model might suit people who were very experienced, because they were already confident and could do their own thinking, but that it was actually probably counterproductive for some students, because they felt they were the only ones struggling with a clinical problem. So we introduced group supervision. I think again that also came from the arts therapy supervision groups that we had at Fulbourn – and I do remember that when you [ER] joined the team, and you became pathway leader, you placed a great emphasis on students helping each other and being responsible, just in their day-to-day working together, which I think again was implicit in the work experience I'd had, but somehow hadn't translated enough into training students. I think that's something that we now do very well at Anglia, and it's crucial. I think you introduced that both on a practical level, in terms of sort of housekeeping, and just people being generally mindful

of each other, but also through the idea that students can really help one other. Everyone's thinking is as important as everyone else's. I am sure that's going on in the experiential groups, but it's now actively fostered in the day-to-day culture of the student group.

Yes, a kind of community model and an important developmental need.
To be able to help one another, people need to be quite mature; any working group also has to face things like competition, and failures of empathy, and the attacks on linking that can happen.

Yes. And in terms of students actually being taught, what's your view now about what sort of group work input there should be? I am thinking very practically now: what should be in the curriculum? Have we got it right at the moment?
Well, I think we could be more explicit about it. I think this book will help, and I think your first book [Davies and Richards 2002] has helped a lot. I think that sometimes students don't realise that they're learning about clinical work through being in a supervision group, although in fact they're learning enormously from each other's work. But what also gets lost sometimes is the idea that they could get to a deeper musical understanding through linking their case experience with their academic work.

We should be getting them to read plenty of theory?
Yes. But I think there is a problem at the moment, and perhaps it originated in the Thatcher era, with the idea of the individual being so much focused upon and people being so out for themselves and gaining material things; the whole capitalist culture hasn't helped the emphasis on group work. So I think it's a complicated picture at the moment, where there's a lot of scepticism about how useful it is for people to sit round and be together. On the other hand, there's a huge 'arts for health' agenda, which is saying that to join a choir and be together and make music is paramount, and it's very healthy.

At the same time, there's also the fact that NHS trusts are very financially constrained these days. It may suit them very well to put patients together into groups.
Yes. I think on the Anglia course we probably do get it about right, because there are so many different strands. There's a composition assessment, which involves a group process, there are the experiential groups, and there are plenty of workshops. I think we could always be more explicit about tying it all into theory, but that happens in supervision groups and in teaching sessions.

Our interest in this conversation has been in group analytic thinking in music therapy, and there's probably another whole discussion to be had about whether that's finding its way into other traditions, like that of community music therapy, for instance, and how much the thinking behind that is informed by analytic ideas.

Indeed. To stay in a more analytic place for now, there has been some interesting work done about comparing processes in other groups, such as orchestras, with music therapy groups – and there has been some interesting writing using musical metaphors to discuss processes in analytic talking groups. Perhaps among the most interesting things in music therapy groups are those moments on the boundary, when the group moves from words to music. Is it a defence against thinking and against something difficult? Or is it actually getting into something that's more difficult? The therapist's role, in my view, is to try and think about that constantly.

Part 2

Group therapy
A group analytic perspective

Chapter 3

Core concepts in group analysis

What goes on in groups? (Part 1)

Nick Barwick

The principle of interconnectedness

S.H. Foulkes, psychoanalyst and originator of group analysis, challenged psychoanalytic orthodoxy on two major counts. First, in contrast to Freud (1921/1991, 1926), he believed that it was possible to 'do therapy' in groups; that a group was not synonymous with a 'mob' and that, under the right therapeutic conditions, it had a natural capacity to nurture its members and to encourage reflective capacity and the development of thought. Second, he believed that a group was a natural medium in which to facilitate such development because it was within a group – the family embedded as it is within the wider groups of community and culture – that 'individuals' are formed. This socio-historical perspective went counter to the dominant psychoanalytic model of the time which, based on a biological perspective, construed the psyche as being formed not by social context, but by innate sexual and aggressive drives, albeit modified by their encounter with the realities of the external world. Thus, though never relinquishing his psychoanalytic loyalties, Foulkes, in elaborating the founding principles of group analysis, drew on 'analytic' traditions beyond psychoanalysis, in particular 'psychological analysis' – especially the work of Kurt Goldstein – and 'sociological analysis' – especially the work of Norbert Elias.

In studying brain-damaged casualties of the Great War, Goldstein became increasingly aware that 'reductive' biological approaches – where simple causal links were made between symptom and 'localised' brain lesion – were insufficient to explain the complexity of patient behaviour. This led him to champion a holistic approach deeply informed by Gestalt psychology, which Foulkes summarises as, 'No finding to be considered without reference to the whole organism and to the total situation' (1936/1990: 43). Thus, though a 'reductive' approach identifies the source of a brain malfunction in one particular part of the brain, a holistic one leads to an understanding that 'Disturbed function is due to the disturbance of the equilibrium of the total situation' (1948/1983: 2).

Foulkes adopts a neurological metaphor to describe how, in a therapy group, each individual is a 'little nodal point' in a 'communicational network' (of people rather than neurons). Each contribution an individual makes not only gains fuller meaning when read against the context of the dynamic network of relationships in which it is made – the 'total situation' – but may be understood as an expression of the communications and/or lack of communications at work within the dynamic system-as-a-whole. This understanding allows Foulkes to re-frame individual psychological disturbance as an expression of disturbed interpersonal processes. Thus, though 'disturbance' may be 'embodied in a particular patient, [it] is in fact the expression of a disturbed balance in a total field of interaction which involves a number of different people' (Foulkes and Anthony 1965/1984: 54).

Elias's sociological perspective further challenges the 'false dichotomy' between 'individual' and group/'society', arguing that individuals can only be understood, indeed only exist, in the context of their 'interdependencies' with each other, as part of networks of social relations, or 'figurations'. Indeed Elias (1939/2000) describes how 'the civilizing process' defines the very nature of individual psychic structure. We are social to the very core.

What we may think of as nature is in fact nurture, though not necessarily of a nurturing kind. This is so because the concept of figuration is not only about interdependence but about function and coercion and therefore about power. Both individuals and groups are interdependent because each fulfils a need for the other. They serve some function. What function they serve depends on the resources available and who has control of them. In effect, the nature of interdependence leaves each party 'capable of exercising some form of reciprocal constraint' (Quintaneiro 2004).

Drawing on Elias, Foulkes states:

> each individual – itself an artificial, though plausible abstraction – is basically and centrally determined, inevitably, by the world in which he lives, by the community, the group, of which he forms a part. . . . the old juxtaposition of an inside and outside world, constitution and environment, individual and society, phantasy and reality, body and mind and so on, are untenable. They can at no stage be separated from each other, except by artificial isolation.
>
> Foulkes (1948/1983: 10)

Fusing Goldstein's notion of a 'network of neurons' with Elias's 'social network'/ 'figuration', Foulkes suggests the group is 'the essential frame of reference in psychology' and that

> the individual is inevitably a fragment shaped dynamically by the group in which he first grew up. . . . a piece of a jig-saw puzzle . . . When you take this individual fragment out of its context, it is shaped and formed, or deformed, according to the place it had and the experiences it received in this group. The first group is normally the family. This family, willy-nilly, reflects the culture to which it belongs and in turn transmits the cultural norms and values.
>
> Foulkes (1974/1990: 275)

What is so powerful here, at an ethical, philosophical and political level, is the notion of shared responsibility for mental health:

> Ultimately it would mean that the whole community must take a far greater responsibility for outbreaks of disturbing psychopathology generally. There is therefore a very specific defensive interest at play in denying the fact of the interdependence which is here claimed; the cry 'but each is an individual' and 'surely the mind is a matter for the individual' means, in this sense, 'each for himself, I am not to blame for what happens to the other person, whether he is obviously near to me, or whether I am involved in concealed ways, or even quite unconsciously.
>
> (1973/1990: 225)

In contrast, Foulkes states, 'Neurosis is not a disease, but arises from problems which concern everybody' (1964: 296). In this light, a group analytic group, representing a microcosm of society, becomes not only an economically pragmatic method of delivering therapy but a preferred method too, for

> if people live from birth on as inter-relational open entities with open valences of bonding, and if individuals are thoroughly socialized and individualized at the same time, and if, during this process, they are liable to produce psychopathological conditions, then we *not only may, but must*, assemble them in a therapeutic group in order to treat them.
>
> Lavie (2005: 520)

In short, 'By the crowd they have been broken, by the crowd they shall be healed' (Marsh 1933).

What is a group analytic psychotherapy group?

Building upon the principle of interconnectedness, Foulkes elaborates several core concepts to describe group analytic theory. Grappling with processes of immense complexity, these descriptions tend to be more 'metaphoric' than precise. For group analysts, this has been a source of both frustration and inspiration, prompting many to draw upon diverse fields, from within and outside psychoanalysis, in search of greater clarity.

Foulkes was not always appreciative of these efforts. Thus only after his death, in 1976, did the full fervour of this eclectic project thrive. As it did so, the application of group analysis widened beyond the psychotherapy group to include median and large groups, organisational consultancy and conflict resolution. Here, however, our focus is the psychotherapy group and the phenomena, described by Foulkes and elaborated by others, at work within it.

Slow open and time-limited groups

The classic group analytic group is a *slow open group*. 'Open' refers to changing composition; members join, members leave. 'Slow' refers to the pace at which these 'beginnings' and 'endings', 'births' and 'deaths' occur. In this 'slow open' way, the group builds a complex family, social and cultural history, which is different from – but resonant with – each member's own family, social and cultural history.

Often, for pragmatic reasons, time-limited group analytic groups are also run. Here, usually, everyone starts and finishes together. The more limited the time, the more limited/focused will be the group's aims and, most likely, the more homogenous the group and the problems presented.

Size

Foulkes recommends a group of seven or eight, plus 'the conductor'. (The conductor is the group analytic term for therapist.) A larger group tends to prompt greater, often annihilatory, anxieties. Intimacy is also often more inhibited and the opportunity for self-presentation reduced. Too small a group, however, pressures the therapist into being more active; less able to allow group dynamics to unfold and the group to do the work. Indeed, certain dynamics, for example those around conflict and difference, may feel riskier or harder to explore. Further, absences threaten group identity when numbers are few.

The stranger group

The classic group analytic group, unstructured in its approach (i.e. without predetermined agenda or rules of engagement), meeting once or twice weekly for ninety minutes, is a *stranger group*. This means members do not know or meet each other outside the group. Any such encounter is a *boundary incident*.

Boundary incidents are not necessarily anti-therapeutic. Discussed in the group, they can provide important opportunities for learning. Unchecked, however, they lead to psychic leakage, depleting the group's life-blood. Secret, they promote sub-groupings that undermine trust in confidentiality and the group's capacity to contain.

On rare occasions, therapists meet members one-to-one. Such meetings demand careful thought regarding what they mean to individual and to group. Opportunities for exploring feelings arising out of such events need to be made.

Composition, cohesion, coherence and integrative-analytic momentum

Foulkes recommends *heterogeneous* groups – '"a mixed bag" of diagnoses and disturbances' (1965/1984: 66). Nevertheless, he recommends no one should be in an isolated position – for example, one young person in a group of older people, one black person in an all-white group, one heterosexual in a group otherwise all gay. Further, the more vigorous the diversity, the more the need for one variable in common. Behind these seemingly conflicting guidelines is an appreciation that, whilst the foundations of self are laid in the experience of safety gained through an encounter with sameness, the development of self, of identity, grows out of an encounter with difference.

Sometimes, the principle of sameness/safety/integration takes precedence over the principle of difference/exploration/analysis. For example, group analysts run groups for women, the elderly, those with eating disorders, those who have experienced torture, those who have suffered abuse. Such homogeneity (be it in terms of social grouping, diagnosis, personality structure and/or life-history/ experience) can promote *cohesion* – a sticking together, or 'bonding' vital to a basic sense of safety without which no exploratory work can be done. The experience of sharing similar experience helps break down feelings of isolation and reduce feelings of shame and abnormality.

Some time-limited groups, in efforts to promote sharing, make establishing safety their main aim. Nonetheless, for any group, it is important to remember that sameness is an illusion, even if, at first, a vital one. To reach its therapeutic potential in terms of interpersonal learning, a group must relinquish sameness and, though valuing similarity, work with difference. Otherwise, cohesion becomes a defensive posture with impermeable boundaries within which difference is expunged. In contrast, the group engaged with both similarity and difference, experiences *coherence* (Pines 1985a/1998) – 'a mindful . . . unity: an aesthetic achievement reached through the reflective and resonant interaction of different parts' (Barwick 2004: 132).

Development

Progression from cohesive to coherent group states is a useful way of thinking about group development. Slow open groups in particular, but time-limited groups too, are susceptible to regressive forces, so such development tends to be oscillating and/or cyclical rather than linear, despite a hoped-for growing capacity for coherence and containment over time. This acknowledges that group analytic groups develop through both integrative and analytic forces: the former bringing people and aspects of people together; the latter, separating out, taking apart. Integrative work precedes analytic work; analytic work is used in the service of integration (Foulkes 1964: 57).

Particularly in closed and/or time-limited groups more linear developmental patterns are observable. For example, a new group, concerned with boundaries and searching for structure, goals and dependence on a leader is focused on 'orientation' (Bennis and Shepard 1956; Yalom 1985). This is followed by 'conflict' over norms, authority and control before a more mature state of 'coherence' is achieved. This matches Tuckman's (1965) group-stage summary: *forming, storming, norming* and *performing*.

In group analytic groups, developmental *tasks* – for each individual joining and for the group as a whole – rather than *stages,* describe the process better. For example:

- *Engagement.* The individual/group struggles with anxiety about being involved in a new situation. Boundary issues, confidentiality and issues of safety predominate.
- *Authority.* Tension about group norms, disclosures and who is confident or not are focused upon.
- *Intimacy.* Questions of trust, attachment and affiliations become core.
- *Change.* Group trust grows; so does self-disclosure. Greater self-exploration allows greater recognition of difference and greater individuation.
- *Termination.* Reflection on changes inside/outside the group are characteristic. What has been 'generalised'? What has not?

adapted from Schlapobersky and Pines (2009)

Core psychoanalytic processes at work in groups

Foulkes suggests three core aspects of psychoanalysis – the unconscious, free association and transference – are equally valid in group analysis. However, even these take on modified forms.

The unconscious

For Foulkes, as for Freud, making the unconscious conscious is core to therapeutic work. Whilst for Freud, though, the unconscious is biological, a bundle of instincts (id), Foulkes broadens this perspective:

> the group-analytic situation, while dealing intensively with the unconscious in the Freudian sense, brings into operation and perspective a totally different area of which the individual is equally unaware ... the individual is as much compelled and modelled by these colossal forces as by his own id and defends himself as strongly against their recognition without being aware of it ... One might speak of a social or interpersonal unconscious
>
> Foulkes (1964: 52)

The social unconscious refers to the *constraints*[1] of social objects (Hopper 2001; Hopper & Weinberg 2011) – socio-cultural communicational arrangements – that have been internalised and of which the individual is 'unaware'. The way such constraints affect us can be seen in the way language influences thinking. For example, if we have a word for something we are more likely to see it – certainly to see it more quickly. Further, the connotations the word has colours the way we see it. Since language is a socio-cultural construct, it carries certain assumptions and prejudices specific to the culture of construction. Hence, to enter into language is to have language (and culture) enter into us: to have our perception shaped by socio-political forces of which we are largely unaware.

For example, Dalal (2002) notes how 'black' in modern Britain has many more negative than positive connotations. This seems 'natural' – black being the colour of the dangerous dark. Yet such connotations are neither asocial nor ahistorical. Indeed, in early seventeenth-century England, positive connotations of black were much more common, 'black' suggesting the exotic more than the illicit or bestial. By the turn of the eighteenth century, however, a marked rise in *denigration* occurs; a change coinciding with colonial expansion. Could it be that the 'denigration' of 'black' became a way of dehumanising non-Christian cultures, so managing, in the wake of our exploitations, European guilt and shame? Such conscious and unconscious linguistic manipulation quickly becomes embedded – expressing a social unconscious that constrains thought in generations to come.

Understandably, we experience resistance to becoming aware of such constraints, partly because we are so caught up in them, partly because the concept compromises the notion of 'free will' (a narcissistic blow), partly because of the guilt awareness exposes us to and partly because society achieves a certain functional stability by being constrained in this way, even when that stability is particularly disadvantageous to the development of some individuals and sub-groups within it.

An appreciation of the social unconscious makes available for analytic scrutiny not only unconscious processes within people but between people and through people. The latter takes the form of 'assumptions' (what is taken for granted and natural in society), 'disavowals' (disowning knowledge or social responsibility for things), 'social defences' (what is defended against by projective mechanisms) and 'structural oppression' (the control of power and information by competing social interests so that awareness is restricted) (Brown 2001).

Dalal (2001) takes issue with the dual model of unconscious – one individual/biological and one social – proposed by Brown (2001) and others. This model, Dalal (1998) argues, follows 'orthodox Foulkes' (one constrained by Freud) rather than 'radical Foulkes' (Foulkes informed by Elias) who proffers a different perspective:

> [the] group, the community, is the ultimate primary unit of consideration, and the so-called inner processes in the individual are internalizations of the forces operating in the group to which he belongs.
> Foulkes (1971/1990: 212)

In effect, 'the things that look like the instincts – the so-called natural ways of behaving – are internalizations of group forces . . . the id itself is acculturated' (Dalal 2001: 543).

Free association

Free association is a fundamental method, in individual psychoanalysis, of accessing the unconscious. The assumption is all lines of thought lead to what is significant – 'the logic of association' being a form of 'unconscious thinking' (Bollas 2008: 21) – except where there is 'resistance'. In group analysis, free association becomes 'group association' or 'free-floating discussion' and refers to thoughts communicated *between* members. As Foulkes comments, 'We now treat association as based on the common ground of unconscious *instinctive understanding* of each other' (1964: 4). Indeed, 'the conversation of *any* group could be considered in its unconscious aspects as the equivalent of free association' (p. 117), though such association is most prevalent in groups, which, like the group analytic group, are unstructured and have no 'occupation' (no explicit focus/task). Indeed, at times, such associations can be particularly rapid, as if capping each other. Foulkes refers to these events as 'chain phenomena'.

Transference

A contemporary understanding of transference combines both 'whole object' and 'part object' perspectives. Whole object transference refers to figures from the past – for example, mother, father, siblings – and a person's experience of them, unconsciously transferred to the present, thus strongly colouring that person's experience of 'new' relationships. Part object transference refers to the fact not only that our experience of present relationships is unconsciously informed by our experience of past relationships but that those past relationships in themselves are coloured by our projections – split off and denied, because unacceptable, aspects of ourselves we assign to others and parts of others – for example, our own aggression. In effect, often what we see in others is what we find it difficult to see in ourselves.

Transference and its interpretation is core to the work of individual psychoanalytic psychotherapy. Foulkes notes how the group analyst is always a Transference figure (capital 'T' denoting transference to the conductor) and that the Transference is likely to be strongly coloured by past authority relations. However, generally he is wary of encouraging the Transference or indeed placing its interpretation at the heart of the group analytic process (see Chapter 5). To do so is to cultivate a dyadic relationship – therapist–patient, therapist–group – which fails to utilise the group's broader life, including multiple transferences (small 't' denoting transferences to other group members) characteristic of the group analytic approach.

T/transferences tend to be seen more vividly in a group and negative Transferences, because of safety in numbers, more freely voiced. Oedipal T/transferences are just such a case in point. Members constantly encounter triadic relationships in which possession of and exclusion from 'the gaze' of another is key. Indeed, individuals can experience, in the here-and-now of the group, whole past patterns of functioning rooted in their family network, just as they can more recent communicational networks such as playgroups, classes, workgroups. Further, a common transference is to the group-as-a-whole as mother.

In addition to multiple individual T/transferences, multiple group T/transferences are also evident. The group T/transferences are collective and often usefully contextualised by the notion of group-as-a-whole development. For example, when a group reaches a certain 'developmental stage', it flexes its muscles, asserting its own authority. Sometimes referred to as the 'barometric event' (Bennis and Shepard 1956), the group Transference can be seen as being to the tribal father whose authority is challenged and must be overcome if it is to be incorporated and the group to 'come of age'.

Group transference to individuals, Foulkes (1964) refers to as 'personification'. Here, a group member may be seen by the group as personifying certain characteristics – the result of collective projections. For example, in a group fearful of loss of control, one member may be identified as personifying uncontrolled aspects of the group. Similarly, in a group assailed by persecutory guilt arising, for example, from surfacing aggression, one person may become identified as aggressor, around whom the whole group carefully treads. Individuals are both coerced into playing these 'parts' as well as often unconsciously drawn to them – what Bion (1961) refers to as 'valency'.

Group members may unconsciously co-create situations belonging to present and/or past wider social, cultural and political contexts (Hopper 2007). Thus feelings of helplessness and loss – perhaps residues from socio-cultural conflicts and traumas transmitted across generations – can forcefully re-emerge within a group (Volkan 2001; Hopper 2003a, 2003b). These types of group transferences are likely to be more prevalent in certain homogenous groups – such as a group of people who have experienced torture and/or persecution – but may be co-created by group members when relevant to a particular member or members within it.

It is not any single Transference then but the web of T/transferences in its entirety that is core to group analysis since it is the 'evolving context of the group' that gives its members an opportunity to 'transcend and transform these powerfully laid down early patterns' (Pines 1985a/1998: 63). Foulkes calls this 'ego-training in action' (1964: 82) – a training based on 'an ongoing corrective interaction with others' (Pines 1985a/1998: 63).

Note

1 Hopper (2003a) clarifies that 'constraint' implies not only 'limitation' but 'facilitation'. For example, the constraints of the sonnet form can facilitate expression.

Chapter 4

Core concepts in group analysis
What goes on in groups? (Part 2)

Nick Barwick

Group-specific processes and phenomena

In addition to the three 'tools' – the unconscious, free association and transference – adopted from psychoanalysis, Foulkes describes several group-specific processes and phenomena.

The matrix

The concept of the 'matrix' epitomises the principle of interconnectedness. Foulkes describes it as 'the hypothetical web of communication and relationship' (1964: 292). He also refers to it as 'the network of all individual mental processes, the psychological medium in which they meet, communicate and interact' (1965/1984: 26). These two metaphors proffer different associations: the former, entanglements, traps; the latter movement, connections. Further, matrix's Latin root, *mater*, means 'mother', whilst the OED defines it as: 'the uterus or womb', 'a place or medium in which something is bred, produced, or developed'. What then is born out of the matrix? What is caught in its web? What develops amidst its connections? It is the individual 'conceived of as a nodal point' and an 'open' rather than 'closed system' (Foulkes 1964: 70). The individual, however, is not passive, for though processes in the matrix pass 'right through all individuals' like 'x-rays', 'each elaborates them and contributes to them and modifies them in his own way' (1973/1990: 229).

Foulkes also refers to the individual as a 'fragment' of a group, 'a piece of a jigsaw' (Foulkes 1974/1990: 275). The first jigsaw of which he is a part is his family (itself, of course, a part of the larger multi-dimensional jigsaws of community, culture and history). Thus the patient brings to the group his *personal group matrix*: an 'individual' mind forged in relation to his group of origin and therefore, in a profound way, an expression of it. Yet as the group develops, a new matrix, formed from the interweaving personal matrices, develops too. This *dynamic matrix* becomes the background against which each individual communication can be understood. Each personal story, each interaction, comes to have a group meaning as well as personal one. It expresses something on behalf of the group as well as something on behalf of the individual.

To these two matrices, Foulkes adds a preceding third: the *foundation matrix*, 'based on the biological properties of the species, but also on the culturally firmly embedded values and reactions' (1975a/1986: 131). Since, 'even a group of total strangers ... share a fundamental mental matrix' (1973/1990: 228), it follows that, 'What we traditionally look upon as our innermost self, the intrapsychic against the external world, is thus not only shareable, but is in fact already shared' (Foulkes 1975b: 62).

Elaborations of the foundation matrix include the 'social matrix' (Burruth 2008) – which recognises that group therapy boundaries are permeable to past and present societal, political and cultural events (Ettin 1993; Stone 2001) and that out of different socio-political environments different psyches are formed – and the more 'mystical', Jungian-influenced perspectives articulated by, for example, Powell (1994) and Zinkin (1998):

> As the group progresses, the members have a growing experience of being connected in their ultimate unity; not just their own unity as a group but a sense of this unity reflecting some ultimate reality which goes far beyond their small circle.
>
> Zinkin (1998: 193)

Powell, noting how an ideology of individualism easily overlooks even our more obvious literal interconnections (such as our immersion, when we sit together in a group, in each other's electromagnetic fields) weaves together analytical psychology and modern physics to argue a metaphysical *and* a physical basis to human interconnectedness:

> Even within the ambit of our universe, events are not related in a linear fashion but form a matrix in space and time in which everything is intimately connected to everything else (the 'holoverse').
>
> Powell (1991: 312)

Whether or not such speculations are of clinical use, at the very least the concept of the matrix continues to convey a powerful understanding of 'individuals as well as of society as *units consistently under construction by communication*' (Scholz 2003: 551). Further, by identifying different matrices, Foulkes alerts us to the '*different time rhythms*' of different types of 'crowd'. The rhythm of change in the foundation matrix (a matter of biological and cultural evolution) is 'slow' whilst the personal matrix, though naturally conservative – preferring to maintain even a difficult psychic status quo – is, potentially, relatively rapid. Most rapid and least conservative is the dynamic matrix and it is within the more fluid, translatable communications of this matrix that the preset jigsaw fragment of the individual is most effectively challenged to change. Further, as individuals do change, so does the dynamic matrix to which they belong. This helps develop greater group coherence and an enhanced capacity to contain. Thus the 'web' becomes 'womb', in which the individual alternately submerges and struggles to emerge, 'strengthened', 're-defined' and 'revitalised' (Roberts 1983).

Location and the 'group mind'

Describing the group matrix, Foulkes (1964) comments:

> Looked at in this way it becomes easier to understand our claim that the group associates, responds and reacts as a whole. The group as it were avails itself now of one speaker, now of another, but it is always the transpersonal network which is sensitized and gives utterance or responds. In this sense we can postulate the existence of a group mind in the same ways as we postulate the existence of an individual mind.
>
> Foulkes (1964: 224)

The notion of 'group mind' is not welcomed by all. Can a group really have a mind when it does not have a brain (Hopper, 2001)? As Weinberg (2007) notes, however, the term does not suggest groups have brains but rather shared hidden motives, myths and defences that guide behaviour. The concept of 'group mind' thus challenges the notion of mind as private individual possession, reframing it as 'interacting processes between a number of closely linked persons, commonly called a group' (Foulkes 1973/1994: 224).

Location is an aspect of 'group mind'. It refers to a group phenomenon where 'interacting processes' emerge as a communication from an individual or set of individuals. This is true even of what is often considered to be the epitome of intrapsychic material, the dream; thus Foulkes's maxim: 'Every dream told in the group is the property of that group' (1964: 127).

Recognising the phenomenon of location makes what is located in the individual (or sub-group) available as a resource (even if, initially, a disturbing one) for the whole group. This promotes psychic development in both individual(s) and group. If location is not acknowledged, however, the individual(s) in whom an aspect of 'group mind' is located will begin to lose psychic flexibility, adopting instead (by dint of past and present group pressures) particular 'roles' – the carer, the victim, the patient, the aggressor. When qualities experienced by the 'group mind' as particularly unacceptable become not only located but more permanently lodged in an individual, *scapegoating* occurs.

Resonance

For Foulkes, the group-specific phenomenon of resonance 'threw new light on the question: how is it possible that the group context produces a shared life from a modality usually conceded only to the "inner" mental life' (1977/1990: 299). Foulkes and Anthony (1965/1984) originally describe resonance as individuals 'reverberating' to some 'common stimulus' – a comment, an absence, a conflict, a dream – 'in a manner specific to the stage [of development] to which they belong' or 'key' to which they are 'attuned':

> These individual vibrations ... create a sort of contrapuntal effect. The overtones add a peculiar richness to a group life occasioning cross-currents of argument, surprise, incredulity, opposition, and interest. It is as if a player, habituated to the narrow range of a single instrument, was suddenly and unexpectedly confronted with a symphonic extension of his little theme.
>
> Foulkes and Anthony (1965/1984: 166)

Resonance to the 'common stimulus' might be expressed verbally, but equally in any number of ways: behaviour, somatic events, accidents, etc. Always, instinctively, it 'takes into account the unconscious meaning and "wavelength" of the stimulating event' (Foulkes 1977/1990: 299). This helps explain how 'that which is neither realized or realizable for the individual is nevertheless activated by the shared processes in the group' (Thygesen 2008). Further, what may start out as isolated communications, through resonance begin to connect harmonically with yet unconscious group preoccupations, like variations on a still-emerging theme. Such organically developing orchestrations enhance social bonding, for

> There is a feeling of well-being which arises when responses of the other resonate with what is sensed as being the most personal of one's experience. This is the essence of progress in group analysis, the presence of other-resonating persons whose inner processes are made both visible and audible through mirroring and resonance.
>
> Pines (2003a: 512–13)

Foulkes suggests resonance occurs at the 'primordial level of communication'. This level Foulkes associates with the 'collective unconscious' (Jung 1968) – an inherited aspect of the psyche, common to all. Although Foulkes did not elaborate on this association, others have. Thygesen (2008), drawing on both contemporary analytical psychology (Spiegelman and Mansfield 1996; Stein 1995) and contemporary psychoanalysis (Gerson 2004; Ogden 2004; Stern 2004), concludes:

> *Resonance* correlates with the constellation of a common connecting mental field ... a changed, often widened state of mind. A 'tuning in' or 'attunement' to what is unconscious to our 'normal ego-consciousness', namely to the group-matrix, takes place ... In the process, ... a dissolution of boundaries, of resistance and defences happens, so that fantasies, thoughts, imagination, feelings, themes lying latent or hidden in the group's matrix, are brought into conscious reflection.
>
> Thygesen (2008: 80)

Amplification and condenser phenomenon

Condenser phenomena are driven by an associative amplification of resonance in the group and refer to

> the sudden discharge of deep and primitive material ... It is as if the 'collective unconscious' acted as a condenser covertly storing up emotional charges generated by the group, and discharging them under the stimulus of some shared group event.
>
> Foulkes and Anthony (1965/1984: 151)

In the release of such energies – for example through the telling of what is sometimes referred to as a 'group dream' (one told by an individual but clearly having group relevance) – there is always an element of surprise, as resonating aspects of the group suddenly coalesce into shared and shareable meaning.

Communication and translation

Foulkes (1964: 114–115) describes four levels of communication in groups:

- the current level (of 'reality') (e.g. the conductor was absent last week)
- the (whole object) T/transference level (e.g. the conductor is treated as if they were a group member's parent)
- the (part object) projective level (e.g. members split off and project parts of themselves onto and into others)
- the primordial level (drawing on Jung's notion of 'collective unconscious', this is where all find themselves 'gripped by an archetype' (Zinkin 1994: 115).

Part of the group's task is to develop its communicative awareness and range. In this, the composition of the group helps. For example, a group that includes over-rationalising members may be complemented by those with freer access to 'lower' (more deeply unconscious) levels of communication (Foulkes 1957: 260–3). The capacity for individualised divergent communicational sensibilities to be woven together to form a stronger, healthier whole has been continually confirmed in clinical practice.

As well as developing depth and breadth of communication, 'working towards an ever more articulate form of communication is identical with the therapeutic process itself' (Foulkes 1948/1983: 169). 'Articulate communication' can be understood here as communication that *is* understandable and *is* understood. In other words, it has meaning for self and other. Foulkes suggests that what a person brings to therapy is an 'autistic symptom' that 'mumbles to itself secretly, hoping to be overheard' (Foulkes and Anthony 1965/1984: 259). It is 'autistic' because, though lodged in the individual, it is a symptom of a breakdown in the communicational network of origin (the family) from which the individual has then become isolated. The therapy group thus offers a re-contextualising network in which the symptom finds a way of being shared and thus articulated. The communicational process of moving from isolated symptom (closed communication with predictable outcome) to shared problem (open communication in the dynamic matrix of the group with unpredictable outcome) to shareable meaning and shared understanding, Foulkes refers to as *translation*; 'the equivalent of the making conscious of the repressed unconscious in psychoanalysis' (Foulkes 1964: 111).

Group analysis can be described as a way of developing 'dialogue for change' (Brown 1986). Schlapobersky (1994) elaborates this notion by distinguishing three forms of dialogue: *monologue* (speaking alone with or without an audience), *dialogue* (a conversation between two people – his use of the word being more specific than Brown's) and *discourse* (the speech pattern of three or more people). In this 'dramatic' model all speech forms have a place, the movement from one to the next being vital to the therapeutic process. Thus monologue is understood as a form of individual self-expression and self-reflection (as in a soliloquy), dialogue a search for intimacy or for 'a resolution of opposites' and discourse, 'the work of the chorus' (Schlapobersky and Pines 2009: 1360), 'true discourse' being the 'defining attribute of group communication' (Schlapobersky 1994: 212).

Habitual monologuing, however, is likely to be defensive rather than developmental. It may be a form of hallucinatory gratification, obliterating feared absence, loss and the need for other. It may be a way of protecting the self against feared intrusion; abuse. Or it may be evidence of a lack of attuned, rhythmical exchanges in the early mother–infant dyad. Here, the act of giving can become muddled with the act of possession, monologuing becoming a socially deviant effort to make contact by colonising the world (Barwick 2006a). The group's capacity to help shift monologue to dialogue to discourse reflects a shift from narcissism to socialism (Lawrence 2003), from isolation to belonging. It marks a growing willingness 'to take the non-problem seriously':

> there is a period in which an individual's presenting problem is accepted by the group. However, after a while, mysteriously the presenting problem is dropped ... in favour of something which is not the problem, not what the individual patient believed he joined the group to involve himself with – it is dropped in favour of the passionate discussion of and involvement with the shifting roles, relationships and behavioural communications which make up the system of the group itself.
>
> Garland (1982: 6)

Mediated by free-floating and reflective *dialogue*, this shift becomes 'an evolution from *despair* and *impotence* to active *desire and hope*' as the experience 'of being part of an ensemble in which candid and daring communication brings about transcendence of what seemed to be an inescapable hopelessness, helps the group members to develop a new stance towards life' (Tubert-Oklander 2010: 137). Such a stance is defined by a deep valuing of 'true intersubjective relationships' and a deeper empathy and understanding not only of self (what is often referred to as insight) but of others ('outsight'), the two being inextricably bound.

Mirroring

Foulkes likens the small group to a 'hall of mirrors' in which 'an individual is confronted with various aspects of his social, psychological, or body image' (Foulkes and Anthony 1965/1984: 150):

> A person sees himself, or part of himself – often a repressed part of himself – reflected in the interactions of other group members. He sees them reacting in the way he does himself, or in contrast to his own behaviour. He also gets to know himself... by the effect he has upon others and the picture they form of him.
>
> Foulkes (1964: 110)

Although the picture formed by others may, as Foulkes concedes, carry distortions rooted in their own individual neuroses, Foulkes asserts that such distortions 'cancel out'; that is, they compensate for each other so the 'composite reflection approximates to the image obtainable in a normal group' (Foulkes and Anthony 1965/1984: 151). Although this assertion arguably oversimplifies, the recognition of mirrored parts of self proffers important opportunities for identity integration and psychological growth (Foulkes 1964) since, 'looking and being looked at is a fundamental process in personality development, in finding out who one is and who one is not' (Pines 1982/1998: 34).

The mirror phenomenon's therapeutic import has been richly elaborated by Wooster (1983), Zinkin (1983) and, most notably, Pines (1982/1998; 1985b/1998; 2003a). Drawing on the work of Mahler, Winnicott, Lacan, Kohut, Stern and others, Pines explores the mirror metaphor in terms of early developmental self–other interactions. Where deficits have occurred (interactions that have undermined or failed to facilitate identity development) they are ripe for corrective re-encounter. For example, contemporary infant research (Stern 1985) identifies the manner in which a sense of self ('the early psychic matrix') begins to form on the basis of reciprocity of gaze, sound and touch. The child's gestures are given meaning by the mother. So too, with the group:

> The more the group members can see and feel their very experience to be meaningful to the group as a whole, so their basic matrix of self is remobilized and worked through in the new group field.
>
> Pines (1983: 12)

Mirroring can also be seen as a conceptual development of projective identification – where aspects of self-experience are unconsciously pushed into another so the other experiences those projected feelings as if their own. Such projections are rife within a group – an integral part of the communicational process (see above). If such projections can find a containing voice, reflection rather than reaction may ensue. This is often a fraught process in which interpsychic 'use' of each other can easily, without the help of the conductor and of the group, become 'ab-use'. Ideally, the matrix takes up the role of container rather than any individual within it.

The discovery of mirror neurons has offered further support for the group analytic view of the importance of mirroring and of the validity of a social mind. Mirror neurons are brain cells that fire up in response to the activity of others. They register 'perceived behaviour, emotions and intentions of others "as if" one were enacting or experiencing them oneself' (Schermer 2010a: 221; 2010b). They thus allow us to 'recognise' human experience in each other, to 'leap into' the mirror of the other and to respond internally as if the other were the self. In other words, 'individuals attune to one another and represent themselves in and through each other, challenging the premise that minds function in relative isolation' (Schermer 2010a: 222). Instead, the embodied mind/brain is revealed as an open, rather than closed energic system (Damasio 1999), inherently biosocial and inextricably linked to its group context (Cozolino 2006). This new knowledge recasts individuals not as social 'atoms' but as 'reflecting mirrors' of the interpersonal world that surrounds them' (Schermer 2010a: 222). Hence, in a group, in a vital and vitalising sense, 'We do not only reflect each other, we *are* each other, until we begin to sort out our own individual nature and tendencies within the group, what Bollas (1989: 109–13) calls our unique "idiom"' (Schermer 2010a: 224). This is to say that, paradoxically, the individuation process depends upon 'the mirroring self-reflection and self-consciousness that can only occur within a social context' (2010a: 225).

Negative mirroring

Foulkes focuses on the nurturing, empathic aspects of mirroring. Nitsun (1996), however, contrasts such benevolent, developmental, 'communicational' mirroring with 'archaic' mirroring. Based on resonances that never achieve higher levels of articulation, archaic mirroring can quickly lead to 'mimetic engulfment' – a loss of separate identity as a result of an unconscious, *en masse* process of imitation – prompting defensive and/or destructive reactions rather than creative reflections.

Weinberg and Toder (2004) identify a number of negative mirrors:

- *The shrinking mirror*: selective mirroring where difference is eschewed; only one aspect of a member, sub-group or group-as-a-whole is seen, e.g. we are all all-nurturing; you/I are/am completely hopeless.
- *The magnifying mirror*: no selectivity here; early in its maturation, before developing into a sound-enough container, the group encourages everyone 'to let it all hang out'. It then finds itself 'flooded' with affect without the means to deal with the flood.
- *The all-knowing mirror:* no room for complexity or doubt. No tolerance of divergent thinking.
- *Lack of a mirror*: everything is seen in terms of the self. Every utterance collapses into the narcissistic pool – 'I feel like that' – followed, often, by

empty, unconnected silence; until the next isolated, stone-prompted ripple. This points to 'early developmental deprivation ... a lack of primary mirroring' (p. 502) – mirroring in the primary care giver's eyes that helps establish an experience of belonging and worth.

All these mirrorings can be seen as malignant. However, 'malignant mirroring' (Zinkin 1983), usually refers to a specific form of negative mirroring: an aversive reaction between two people, as if each sees in the other some aspect of themselves that is too horrifying and/or shameful to acknowledge. Intensified denial and projection follow. Locked in a terrorised and terrorising gaze based on mutual projective identifications, each participant is both repelled and fascinated by the mirror in which they look. Zinkin identifies malignant mirroring as an interpersonal interaction – between pairs of individuals or sets of individuals. However, the pair thus engaged often also enacts transpersonal dynamics at work in the group involving the same processes of splitting, denial and projective identification.

Triadic mirroring and the 'model of three'

'Observation and self-observation in a social setting' is a crucial therapeutic activity (Foulkes 1948/1983). Foulkes refers to the contribution of the 'observer', in his 'model of three':

> if A and B are two persons between whom this interaction takes place, it would appear to me that the presence of a third person C is required if this interrelationship is to be seen in perspective ... This model, which one might call the *model of three*, is to my mind the simplest elementary model for the understanding of interpersonal relationships. C represents that new third dimension group observation introduces.
>
> Foulkes (1964: 49)

Foulkes does not elaborate greatly upon this model. However, elsewhere, linking this to a contemporary object relations view of the Oedipal situation, I suggest that the development of observational capacity or 'witness-training in action' is a vital aspect of group analytic work (Barwick 2004). The capacity to 'bear witness' is founded upon the capacity to bear exclusion; that is to remain empathically connected to that which one is not entirely a part. This is an important developmental achievement having many psychological ramifications, not least the development of 'a capacity for seeing ourselves in interaction with others and for entertaining another point of view whilst retaining our own, for reflecting on ourselves whilst being ourselves' (Britton 1989: 87). The capacity to witness in this way, Britton refers to as maintaining 'a third position'.

Pines (1982) draws on the story of Perseus to illustrate the need for a perspectival third position in the slaying of personal gorgons. Perseus's journey is into the inner depths of the Psyche, of which the gorgon, Medusa, is symbolic of one 'shadow-oriented' aspect (Diel 1980, cited in Pines 1982/1998). The stony paralysis and consequent demise of those who have previously made the venture can be understood as resulting from an inability to contemplate the objective truth about oneself. Yet the success of the venture is vital to psychic development. Only by facing one's inner demon is the individuation process furthered, the shadow-self integrated, and the creative potential both liberated and controlled. Thus the blood from Medusa's neck gives life to Pegasus, the horse of the Muses, which enables Perseus to continue his psychic quest.

The point is that the gorgon can only be faced with the help of a third, in this instance, Athena's armour, which, polished, becomes a mirror in which Perseus can witness Medusa and, in the witnessing, deal with her. Relating this to the group in which individual members may see mirrored (in other members' interactions with each other), hated and disavowed aspects of their own selves, Pines suggests that what otherwise might lead to 'entranced' or 'entangled' forms of projection – such as malignant mirroring – 'receives a triadic form of mirroring, one at a higher developmental level'. Through this triadic mirroring, 'a benign cycle of projection and introjection is initiated which can often lead to the freeing up of the closed psychic system and thereby to renewed psychic growth' (Pines 1982/1998: 27).

Wooster (1983) suggests malignant mirroring – where there is an absence of a third position – may find its source in deficits in early triangulation experiences. Drawing upon Abelin (1971; 1980) to identify the developmental stage at which the child is forced, by the intrusion of the father, to become aware of exclusion from an imitative, narcissistically-mirroring relationship with his mother, Wooster notes that the child must take up a position as an observer and, in recognising his separateness, enter a shared symbolic realm. This is a realm in which 'reflection begins to replace reaction' (Pines 1982/1998: 30). Indeed, in part, the child learns the capacity to observe and reflect *from* his father. The father, after all, will have experienced exclusion from the 'nursing couple' and will, ideally, not only have tolerated it but, in the early stages, by protecting the mother–child dyad, have actively encouraged it as well. Thus, in addition to being a rival, it is *with* the father that the child must identify. In effect, a 'favourable outcome' to the child's witness-training programme may depend 'on the positive and emulatory aspect of the three-person jealousy inherent in the situation'. This, in turn, is very much informed by the 'father's own capacity to work through his initial jealousy about this intrusive newcomer breaking up the original husband/wife duo' (Wooster 1983: 38). It is the absence of such a 'favourable outcome' that may lead to malignant mirroring.

The intervention in the negative dyadic relationship, then, of the mirror as 'third element', creates the psychological space for dialogue, for the holding of different points of view about the same experience, and for exploration. Where there is no triangulation of space, there is 'no capacity for reflection and for meeting on shared ground'. This means that there can be 'no acceptance of an aspect of self that is reflected in the other and also of the other in the self' (Pines 1982/1998: 34). In the therapy group, if neither party can manage the reflexive activity of witnessing their own interactions, other witnesses – the therapist and other group members – must be called.

Exchange

Exchange is the process of interactive sharing in a group. It is usefully paired with mirroring: the latter implying similarity or sameness; the former difference. And, as Zinkin (1994) states, 'People are helped both by identifying with others and by recognising their differences' (p. 103).

Essentially, what is exchanged is 'information' (Foulkes 1964: 34): 'information' as 'news of difference'; 'differences that make a difference' (Bateson 1979). Constant exposure to reported and enacted different ways of seeing, being and doing can be deeply and productively challenging, producing a liveliness and directness of exchange, particularly in terms of feedback, that is more difficult to envisage in the asymmetrical relationship of the therapy dyad.

Dalal (1998) also emphasises the potentially transformational nature of exchanging 'information':

> Information is another name for what Elias has called knowledge, and ... this is the same as language and thought. Elias's insight was that the state of knowledge is inextricably entwined with the state of the psyche. When this is joined up with Foulkes' notion of communication, we can see how and why speech is potentially a transformational and therapeutic act.
>
> Dalal (1998: 223)

Dalal's metaphor is penetrative, dramatic:

> To speak is one thing, to listen is another. To listen is potentially a very frightening process, because to hear the words of another is literally to let their words and meanings into the self – it is to let a stranger into the home. And once they have entered, who knows where they may go, what havoc they may wreak, or what changes they may precipitate?
>
> Dalal (1998: 223)

Drawing on the analogy of exchange in the early mother–infant relationship, Thornton's metaphor is less so, though far-reaching in its impact nonetheless:

> Exchange in that first relationship is of far more than milk and bodily contacts; there is acknowledgement of feelings and of mutuality in feeling, and there is reciprocal observation.
>
> Padel (1985: 275) cited in Thornton (2004: 312)

In groups then, the vitality of exchange is pre-verbal as well as verbal, having transformative value independent of content. This is not to underestimate the impact of linguistic exchange, only to complement it, for language, as a carrier of 'content', has always had a significant role to play in shaping our experience of ourselves in the presence of others. This is so since 'with language, infants, for the first time, can share their personal experience . . . including "being with" others in intimacy, isolation, loneliness, awe, fear and love' (Stern 1985: 182).

In the group, as feeling states are put into words and exchanged, as difference is encountered, recognised and identified with, as isolating experience is converted into 'exchangeable currency' (Behr and Hearst 2005: 86), the 'shareable universe', inner and outer, expands, giving truth to Merleau-Ponty's (1964) poignant observation: 'I borrow myself from others; man is a mirror for man' (cited in Pines 1985a/1998: 68).

Conclusion: The socialising process

In group analysis, socialisation is a core therapeutic factor:

> The patient is brought out of his isolation into a social situation in which he can feel adequate . . . he can feel understood as well as show understanding of others. He is a fellow being on equal terms.
>
> Foulkes (1964: 33)

Socialisation is about feeling part of the human world; a belongingness achieved by gaining insight *and* outsight. Related to these is an appreciation that change and growth are rooted not only in 'regressive behaviour' – what others can do for oneself – but in 'progressive behaviour' – what one can do for others.

Socialisation is also about understanding something of how we become who we are; how identity is formed and re-formed within and by the matrices *to* which we contribute and *of* which we are a part. As later group analysts note, the 'socialising process' in a group is not always as benign as Foulkes suggests and the health of the 'norm' with which, Foulkes argues, the individual in the group is gradually brought in line, needs itself to be available to analytic scrutiny. Nonetheless, the principle of releasing the individual from isolation – that is, promoting in him the capacity for empathy as well as the experience of being empathised with – and of introducing him, through reflecting on interpersonal experience, to the principle of interconnectedness, remains central to the experientially based psycho-social venture that is group analysis.

Chapter 5

Core concepts in group analysis
What does the conductor do?

Nick Barwick

Group analysis is 'a form of psychotherapy *by* the group, *of* the group, including the conductor' (Foulkes 1975a/1986: 3). The group is thus the agent of change; the conductor simply part of the group. And yet, the conductor is also different. His very name makes him so; someone who

> sets a pattern of desirable behaviour ... puts emphasis on the 'here and now' ... promotes tolerance and appreciation of individual differences. ... represents and promotes reality, reason, tolerance, understanding, insight, catharsis, independence, frankness, and an open mind for new experiences.
> Foulkes (1964: 57)

As conductor, he contributes powerfully to the development of a 'group analytic culture'; a culture in which radical reconfiguration of identity can occur.

The conductor and authority

Foulkes takes the term 'conductor' from Theodor Adorno. Adorno's research into the fluctuating authority in the orchestra–conductor relationship offered Foulkes a blueprint for understanding the therapist's authority in relation to the psycho- therapy group; broadly speaking, one which assumes a more active role early in the group's life – modulating tempo, attending to individual instruments, linking instruments and sections of instruments together, interpreting the score – and works towards a 'decrescendo' of such activity over time.

Unsurprisingly, in the context of fascism, Foulkes was wary of a group's tendency to conform to the conscious and unconscious beliefs of a leader (or Führer).[1] Indeed, Foulkes saw the 'correction' of authority relations (internalised in the superego) as a key therapeutic task. The manner in which the conductor 'leads' the group thus becomes a significant factor in facilitating this task.

Foulkes identifies two roles for the conductor, each requiring the adoption of a 'position'. As 'administrator' (the person responsible for establishing and maintaining the structure of therapy) the position is of 'executive authority'. As 'therapist' (the person facilitating process and interpreting content), it is of 'expert authority', shaping the therapeutic culture of the group (Hutchinson 2009). In the executive position, wielding a non-transferable 'power over others', the conductor must manage a number of challenges to his authority. By responding with genuine curiosity as well as non-punitive firmness, he contributes significantly to the internalisation of a modifying experience of authority relations; that is, to a maturing of the superego.

In contrast, expert authority *is* transferrable; its transfer being one of the conductor's aims. The process is analogous to 'weaning'. Initially, the conductor accepts the group's projections – the power, the 'father complex' (Foulkes and Anthony 1965/1984: 119). Yet he does so only to relinquish it; 'to change from being a leader *of* the group to being a leader *in* the group' (Pines et al. 1982: 156). Since a leader's power is based largely upon projections of parts of the superego of those 'following', its transmission involves a reintrojection of a modified superego achieved through '*transference analysis in action*' (Foulkes 1975a/1986: 112). Describing the conductor's active contribution to the decrescendo in the therapist's expert authority and the accompanying crescendo in the group's, Foulkes also draws on a less clinical analogy: 'The conductor,' he says, 'digs his own grave' (Foulkes 1964: 62).

Dynamic administration

The conductor attends to three aspects of group life: *structure*, *process* and *content* (de Maré 1972). Structure describes the 'architecture' in which the group's interpersonal life is housed: the analytic setting, the organisational setting and membership itself. Process refers to fluctuations of emotion and experience within the group: the 'business of relating and communicating' (Schlapobersky and Pines 2009: 1355). Content refers to verbal and non-verbal events: emergent narratives, themes and their development. As dynamic administrator, structure is the focus of attention.

The analytic and organisational settings

The analytic setting includes the room and its contents (chairs, table, etc.) and the boundaries (time, frequency) in which the physical setting is placed. The room and its contents – ideally, identical seats arranged in a circle with a small table[2] at its centre – can be understood as an extension of the conductor's body, of his 'holding' capacity. Thus, the room's constancy, apt quietness and freedom from external impingements help cultivate a sense of dependability and safety. Further, by keeping the setting relatively constant, the significance of any changes that do occur becomes available for analytic scrutiny.

Attending to the relationship between the wider organisation and the analytic setting is also vital. This is to acknowledge that the group meets in the context of a network of social interdependencies, the neglect of which risks, at best, de-stabilising impingements on the *boundaries* of the analytic setting, at worst, the dissolution of the group itself.

Boundaries, boundary incidents and principles of conduct

Preparing members for the group is likely to enhance group functioning and reduce drop-out (Slavendy 1993). As part of this preparation, the conductor introduces each member, prior to joining the group, to certain 'principles of conduct' (Foulkes 1975a/1986). These help regulate the boundaries of the setting:

- discretion (what is presented in the group remains in the group)
- regularity and punctuality
- notification of absences
- payment of fees (if the work is private)
- no contact outside the group
- abstinence (to refrain from behaving in ways that reduce tension or distract attention from emotional content)

That these are principles rather than 'rules' acknowledges that any transgression (boundary incident) requires analytic interest more than enforcement. Handled well, such incidents usually offer opportunities for development.

Nevertheless, the conductor must respond with firmness as well as curiosity. Though there can be no useful imposition of principles, principles are, nonetheless, vital to group analytic culture. Championing them in non-punitive but resolute ways requires the conductor to feel relatively confident about his own internalised authority relations and, retaining executive authority, to remain in role. In this light, though Foulkes's recommendation that, following the session, the conductor keep an attendance register may appear schoolmasterly, it helps highlight emergent patterns, as does recording who sits next to whom, including the conductor.

The conductor also needs to attend to what might seem more benign 'boundary incidents'. For example, should a member offer to help ready furniture prior to the group, the conductor must remember he is a 'Transference figure' and that any such offer has meanings that should not be lost to the emerging matrix of the group. Similarly, after a group, should a member approach the conductor about some 'private' matter, the conductor must encourage them to bring the matter to the group. Indeed, all communications (conversations, emails, texts, telephone messages) that take place between members (including the conductor) outside the group belong to the same network as those that take place inside the group. It follows, if the group's matrix is not to be depleted, all need to be made available *to* the group.

Challenges to the physical setting – members rearranging chairs, shifting the table – can also occur. Whether to confront these concretely – for example, by returning a moved table – or whether, noting them, to wait until session material offers an opportunity for a more reflective intervention, is a matter of clinical judgement. Whichever the approach, both holding the boundary and making such communications available for analytic scrutiny are essential for group safety and development.

Selection

> Group composition is the therapist's first and most enduring contribution to the group, for its membership will determine the outcome of therapy.
> Schlapobersky and Pines (2009: 362)

In assessing membership, the conductor keeps three things in mind: suitability for group therapy, for this particular group, for this particular group at this particular time. These last two aspects concern patient 'fit': matching individual with group resources and needs. For example, if the prospective group is mature (that is, not overly dependent, reasonably capable of containing disturbance without feeling overwhelmed and reasonably reflective) introducing a member with borderline personality disorder may be mutually beneficial. Having quicker access to unconscious forces, such members can help fuel group momentum. In return, the group can help regulate the intensity of their affective swings. However, if the group is insufficiently mature, interpersonal disturbances provoked are unlikely to benefit either individual or group (Pines 1984/1998).

In terms of general suitability, Foulkes suggests anyone suited for individual psychotherapy is suited for group. Brown (1991) tempers this view but agrees with Foulkes that the ability to communicate in a group is vital. This calls for assessment based on interpersonal skills. Related contra-indicators might be people who are too narcissistic to be capable of identification with other members, too needy to contemplate sharing attention (something often linked with very early traumatic loss/deprivation), are too undifferentiated to withstand the group's emotional currents/storms, have very poor impulse control or hold such rigid belief systems they appear impervious to other perspectives (Behr and Hearst 2005: 65). On the other hand, for some whose attachment patterns can make them wary of the intimacy of a one-to-one relationship or, conversely, have 'a tendency to get overly enmeshed in sticky, clingy and perhaps parasitic transferences in dyads' (Hopper 2006: 555), group therapy may, initially at least, be the treatment of choice.

Schlapobersky and Pines (2009: 1362) offer a useful summary of inclusion and exclusion criteria:

Inclusion:
1 motivation to address personal issues
2 willingness to try and participate
3 some experience of successful relationships

4 some interest in exploring/understanding self
5 some capacity to talk, listen and relate
6 some interest in others
7 some sense that being amongst others might be helpful
8 some ability to sympathise with others' needs and problems
9 some indication of future reliability in attendance

Exclusion:
1 those in acute crisis
2 prior history of broken attendance in therapy
3 major problems of self-disclosure
4 major problems with reality testing (paranoid/psychotic)
5 pathological narcissism
6 difficulties with intimacy generalised into personal distrust
7 defences that rely excessively on denial and disassociation
8 emotional unavailability
9 tendency to be verbally subdued or withdrawn
10 tendency to be hostile and aggressive, verbally or otherwise

For inclusion, prospective members should meet at least four inclusion and no more than four exclusion criteria.

From dyad to group

Selection and preparation usually occur over several one-to-one sessions. Concerned about patient–therapist attachment complicating member–group attachment – the shift from sole to shared 'ownership' of 'conductor–parent' being potentially problematic – some conductors keep one-to-one contact to a minimum. Others, however, see such secure one-to-one attachment as providing an important anchor for the patient negotiating entry into the group.

Of course, just as each new member needs preparation for entry into the group, the established group needs preparation for the entry of a new member. Mature groups may make such preparations themselves, giving time to reflect on hopes, fears and expectations. However, when there is reluctance to do so, the conductor must encourage such reflection (whilst simultaneously noting, with interest, the reluctance shown). Such 'noting' captures how, at certain points, dynamic administration inevitably bleeds into therapeutic activity.

Therapeutic activity

A conductor's therapeutic activity is synonymous with his *interventions*. Interventions generally describe verbal utterances: questions, clarifications, challenges, observations, interpretations. However, they also describe behaviours: gestures, entry in and out of the group, the taking of a particular chair. Indeed, even a conductor's seemingly passive presence is an 'intervention', since his capacity to observe and attune to emotional currents in the group can itself provide significant holding and containing functions. Conversely, a conductor's persistent silence and reserve (one might say 'absent' presence) may be experienced as uncaring, neglectful and threatening.

A conductor's interventions combine 'masculine' and 'feminine' elements – reserve, robustness and penetration associated with the first; empathy, tolerance and receptivity with the second. A Foulkesian perspective – epitomised by the motto, 'Trust the group' – considers a well-constituted group to be naturally creative and nurturing. This has led to an emphasis upon the conductor's complementary 'feminine' function. Consequently, even a conductor's more active interventions are often characterised by 'lightness of touch' or 'a nudge in the right direction'.

The practice of group analysis, however, is littered with casualties – drop-outs, scapegoats, those who have become more disturbed – suggesting group forces far less benign at work. Concepts such as 'the anti-group' (Nitsun 1991; 1996) help describe these more destructive aspects (see Chapter 7); ones which demand, perhaps, more 'masculine', active interventions.

How do conductors intervene?

Research into conductor interventions identify several types (Kennard et al. 1990; 1993) each attending to one of the three aspects of group life – structure, process and content – already described.

Maintenance

Maintenance interventions aim to clarify and/or reaffirm relevant boundaries. Ideally, such interventions arise out of the interpersonal communicational processes of the group. For example, one member expresses anger at another for never being on time; another great concern about a member's absence with no message. However, if the group does not 'intervene', the conductor must, particularly if such boundary incidents are pervasive, suggesting anti-group forces at work.

Open facilitation

Open facilitation aims to promote group 'process' without seeking to influence its direction. It is a 'lubricating activity'. It may take the form of an observation, a clarification or a reflecting back. Whichever the form, there is no conscious hypothesis regarding underlying dynamics or issues but rather a signal of interest in the process of communication itself and in the worth of thinking about what is going on. The conductor may gain the group's assistance in the task of thinking simply by saying, 'I wonder what everyone thinks is happening in the group at this moment.'

Guided facilitation

Guided facilitation is more directional but typically 'light-handed' nonetheless. The conductor, having some hypothesis about what is going on – latent aspects ripe for translation – finds a way of directing the group's attention to it. In effect, he provides a 'stepping-stone' for an individual and/or for the group towards meaning-making.

Interpretation

Foulkes notes that many of the individual contributions members make to the process of free-floating discussion are 'unconscious interpretations' of prior contributions in the group (1968/1990: 181). Organically, this helps develop the meaning-making group culture Pines describes:

> At a deeply unconscious level, as when a person speaks of a symptom, of a difficulty in life, of mental pain or conflict, the response of the other group members can often illuminate the presenting person's unconscious processes. This illumination comes from the authentic knowledge that one person has of another, based upon deep personal involvement in the therapeutic situation.
>
> Pines (1993: 100)

As such 'interpretative' processes unfold – as surface is exchanged for depth, symptoms for meaning, isolation for communication – the conductor's role is essentially one of 'watchful gentleness' (Trevarthen 1977: 337), of 'fundamental unintrusiveness' (Bollas 1987), rather than direct interpretative intervention.

Nevertheless, conductor interpretations – those offering psychoanalytically informed meaning to patients' contributions and interactions where previously either there was no apparent meaning or where the meaning conveyed is different from that suggested – are necessary at times and Foulkes offers some 'guiding lines' as to when and how they should be made:

> Interpretation is called for when there is a blockage in communication. It will be particularly concerned with resistances, including transference. Its form and content should be determined by the ongoing interaction and communication as experienced by the group. For its location and timing the emotion of the patients should be followed.
>
> Foulkes (1975a/1986: 125)

Related to this is his warning against 'plunging interpretations': those that go from surface to primitive depths, stirring such profound anxieties that the patient either responds in an intellectualised manner or ignores the interpretation altogether.

Conductors tend to be sparing in their use of interpretation and, when interpreting, tend to address the group-as-a-whole more than the individual. Such reticence finds its roots in Foulkes's (1975a) aphorism: 'interpretation comes in where analysis fails' – analysis being 'the totality of the work directed at making the unconscious conscious'; 'the establishment of more and more specific meaning by patient exploration' (p. 117). After all, 'in giving an interpretation we do the work which the patient ought to do' (p. 116) – that is, the work of translation.

Comparing the development of the group's capacity to translate with a child learning to speak, Foulkes adds, 'If the child is too readily understood by its parents on an infantile level it will make no effort to increase its mastery of language' (Foulkes and Anthony 1965/1984: 263). Further, conductor-proffered interpretations tend to promote him as primary source of analytic wisdom, intensifying projections of authority whilst simultaneously demoting the authority and creative potential of the group. This does not deny the occasional usefulness of offering a direct interpretation to an individual, particularly if something, despite being near the surface, is not being addressed by the group. If proffered, however, an incomplete interpretation is often preferable. This can prompt group reflections that often have the capacity to take the individual (and the group) far further than the conductor is able to alone.

Transference interpretation

Transference provides immediate, live access to a patient's relational history and/or ways of relating. It is thus one of the most significant dynamics active within the therapeutic situation. So valuable is the information it proffers, individual therapists, with neurotic patients at least, tend to encourage its 'maturation'. In part, such 'transference neurosis' is enabled by the nature of the analytic attitude – generally characterised by a high degree of restraint, reserve and neutrality, be it with an affirmative tone. In its most classical form, this amounts to providing a 'blank screen' on which the patient's projections may be 'thrown' (Freud 1913/2002). Indeed, Kleinians refer to actively 'gathering the transference' (Meltzer 1968) and to transference in therapy as the 'total situation' (Joseph 1985). It is unsurprising then that, in individual therapy, the transference interpretation (in particular one which links through the 'transference triangle' (Malan 1979) the patient's relationship with current others outside the therapy to the therapist and to figures from the past) is seen by most psychoanalytic practitioners as the single most significant mutative intervention a therapist can make (Hobson and Kapur 2005).

Foulkes notes the inevitable significance of the conductor as a Transference figure, particularly with reference to his authority in the early stages of a group. However, rather than 'gathering' such f/phantasies, Foulkes (1975a/1986) advises he 'must avoid becoming too important and must keep to the background', for if he manages to 'minimise his significance', not only will he be in a better position to analyse a patient's projections but 'he will make the group into a more confident and active agent.' Hence, 'The group will learn to rely more on itself and be correspondingly more convinced of the truth of its findings' (p. 111).

The fact that, in a group, the Transference is one among many transferences (see Chapter 3) is another reason the conductor declines to 'gather' it. To do so would be to inhibit fuller development of the matrix (including complex multiple transferences) by giving prominence to the dyad: conductor–patient, conductor–group. Further, though the conductor may, at times, offer interpretations regarding these multiple transferences, much of the time such dynamics are challenged by 'real' responses from group members as part of the process of communication. This encourages a 'corrective family group experience':

> There is a built-in correction of the transference phenomena through the peer relationship in groups. The analyst is trained to let the transference neurosis grow to full bloom. Members of a group are neither trained nor willing to accept such projections . . . and will correct them.
>
> Grotjahn (1977: 14)

For the conductor, a natural outcome of gradually declining aspects of the Transference role is his greater freedom to be himself. Although abstaining from personal disclosure in terms of history or current reality, he has licence to be more spontaneous, more liberal in affective communication and more willing to engage playfully, sometimes humorously, within the matrix of the group.

Though less reserved, the conductor hopes, nonetheless, to monitor rather than enact his own transferences. Even so, such relational purity is unlikely. Although the group will not have access to the conductor's relational context outside the group, they will have access to past and present relations inside. This is enough to prompt observations and hypotheses about the way he relates in the group. Such scrutiny is valid analytic work and, though the conductor must be mindful of whether anti-group or developmental forces motivate, he must also be open to discourse that helps modify authority relations and promotes the growing maturity of the group. In effect, the conductor should be willing to accept and even invite the group's help with his blind spots (Hopper 2006).

Countertransference

To speak of a therapist's 'blind spots' is to highlight the issue of countertransference. Countertransference has a long, complex history. Seen classically as a form of therapeutic contamination (either the analyst's own transference to the patient, or their emotional response (counter) to the patient's transference), the remedy is further analysis for the analyst. Taking a more contemporary 'totalistic' view (Kernberg 1965), though still recognising the importance of being alert to potentially contaminating 'blind spots' (both personal and professional[3]), Prodgers (1991) recasts it as an invasion of the analyst's unconscious by the patient's which, as long as the analyst is not captured, becomes a rich source for understanding the patient's internal world.

In some ways, Foulkes took quite a 'classical' view of countertransference. Invasive, destabilising, he refers to it as a 'Trojan horse' (Foulkes 1958/1990). However, through the concept of resonance, in which the conductor participates as much as any member, Foulkes's view of countertransference is much more totalistic. Indeed, Foulkes goes much further than most analytic models by suggesting the conductor not only should work with such 'communications', helping to translate them into more articulate forms, but should also, at times, offer a form of countertransference disclosure.

The 'best hint' as to whether such disclosure is 'useful or even necessary' is, Foulkes suggests, whether the conductor 'becomes aware that some resistance against communication is located in himself, is involving him if not caused by him' (1975a/1986: 114). This is to take seriously the fact that the conductor is both observer *of* and participant *in* the group. As participant, he is exposed to and penetrated by the interacting processes that constitute the matrix of the group.

Many group analysts draw on object relations thinking when working with countertransference. This describes the process by which denied, split off aspects of self are projected into others so that what is projected is experienced by the other as if it were their own. The conductor's countertransference may thus be understood as an emotional response to (resonance with) these projections. It is the process of containment – making meaning out of what has been projected and re-presenting this in more digestible, knowable form – that brings the patient psychic growth (through reintrojection of the projected aspects) and relief.

Other group analysts draw more on self-psychology and intersubjective theory. Distinguishing between 'conflictual transference' – which defends against the patient's fear of being retraumatised by environmental failure – and 'self-object transference' – the expression of longing for someone to meet developmental needs – countertransference offers the conductor insight into the nature of the need and ways in which it might be addressed.

Drawing on Argelander (1970), Beck (2006) introduces the notion of 'scenic understanding' to the idea of working with the countertransference – 'scenic' referring to dramatic enactments (or reenactments) on a stage. In a group, a particular member's traumatising relationships from the past begin to be reenacted in the here-and-now relationships of the group. Resonance then takes over, helping to find 'a common denominator, a trauma or conflict shared more or less by the whole group' (Beck 2006: 103). The conductor's first job is one of 'scenic observation': a careful watching, from an analytically informed perspective, of the creation of the enactment. 'Scenic experience' quickly accompanies such observation: the conductor's own resonance, his experience of being invaded by the resonances at work in the group as a consequence of the enactment and of being pulled towards a particular way of relating. This needs to be followed by 'scenic intervention': the conductor's description, offered to the group, of 'the roles and attitudes evolving within him/her during this process, and the ideas he/she has in the state of functional regression' (p. 104). Although some group analysts might be wary of too interpretative an intervention, such descriptions may also be offered by way of invitation – part of hermeneutic research in which the whole group may join. Whichever the approach, Beck's summary remarks are unlikely to be contested:

> It is not enough to become nothing but a part of the situation. Also, it is not enough to observe the situation from outside and just think about its meaning. In a therapeutic ego-split, we have to oscillate between being affected by and involved in the situation, and to reflect about what is being enacted.
> Beck (2006: 104–5)

In a group context, although the conductor has the role of therapist, all members work in a therapeutic capacity. Further, since transference and associated projective processes are ubiquitous, each member, as well as the group-as-a-whole, is likely to experience countertransference responses to the interactions within and of the group. Indeed, 'Communication through projective identification is a vital part of group life and often provides an effective pathway for psychological growth' (Rogers 1987: 99). The conductor's job is to encourage a maturing of such primitive communicative methods into more sophisticated forms, such as 'putting it into words'. Since this tends not to happen easily, those finding themselves used as a container for split-off and projected aspects of others will themselves need help (and support) in recognising that this dynamic may be at play. In effect, part of the 'witness training-in-action' already described (see Chapter 4), in its development of a capacity for self-observation and the observation of interactions in which one is involved, can also be seen as a form of 'countertransference training-in-action'.

Why, when (and more about how) conductors intervene

Facilitating communication

The prime reason for intervening is to facilitate 'working towards an ever more articulate form of communication [which] is identical to the therapeutic process itself' (Foulkes 1948/1983: 69); or more accurately, to facilitate the group's capacity for such work. Thus, 'Foulkes' clinical recommendations to the conductor can be summarised as a responsibility for promoting discourse' (Schlapobersky 1994: 228).

Communicational fluidity (promoted and characterised by resonance, communicational mirroring and exchange) enables greater articulateness because it ensures all parts of the communicational network remain part of the whole. Nonetheless, characteristic of a network is that parts do, temporarily at least, become 'mouthpieces' for broader dynamics at play. This becomes problematic only if the communicational current becomes blocked, leaving individuals isolated from social context and their symptoms 'autistic' in that isolation.

Working with resistance

Another way of describing such blockages is 'resistance'. This recasts what otherwise might be construed as accidental as meaningfully, if unconsciously, motivated. Where there are communicational resistances the group seems tardy, reluctant and/or unable to address, the conductor must intervene. Even so, the constructive function of resistance – a means of defending against overwhelming anxiety – must be kept in mind. This helps alert the conductor to the pace and manner of intervention.

Working with resistance to shifting conversations in time-and-place

Group communications may focus on the 'here-and-now' (the present inside the group), the 'here and then' (the past inside the group), the 'there-and-now' (the present outside the group) and the 'there-and-then' (the past outside the group). Without guidance, therapy groups often focus on 'outside' communicational modes. Here, problems are aired, personal narratives shared and strong resonances evoked. However, experience is, of necessity, at one remove. It is *re*called. By contrast, conductors often draw on such narrative experiences to both fuel and shift the focus to the 'inside', particularly the 'here-and-now'. Here, narrative gives way to drama as the group struggles to work in the transference. In this often-turbulent arena, much interpersonal learning may be achieved, since problems brought become recognisable in the immediacy of interpersonal encounter and a corrective recapitulation of early family life is possible.

At times, however, the nature of the communicational blockage prompts the conductor to turn the usual interventional focus on its head. For example, if there has just been a bombing nearby and the group focuses only on the here-and-now, the absence of narrative regarding the wider social matrix alerts the analyst to a de-cathexis – a withdrawal of emotional energy from the 'there-and-now' – about which the conductor needs to alert the group (Burruth 2008).

Working with resistant conversations

All groups have conversations aimed at ensuring 'nothing beneath the surface is disturbed or exposed' (Roberts and Pines 1992: 486). If persistent, the conductor may need to draw attention to these. Nevertheless, 'phatic communion' – 'a type of speech in which ties of union are created by a mere exchange of words' (Malinowski 1923: 314) – can help provide necessary levels of safety and social bonding and should not be lightly dismissed. Further, language's metaphorical nature naturally affords room for the unconscious, even in communication that appears mundane; for example, a group conversation about the dearth of parking as a metaphor for individual concerns about finding room in the group. As Foulkes notes, 'Depth is always there . . . It depends who is looking, who is listening; one need not jump from what is going on to what is behind it' (1974/1990: 280).

More problematic may be conversations which appear probing but focus only on one individual. Although taking the guise of therapeutic endeavour, the conductor must keep in mind what is being located in the individual – need, vulnerability, inadequacy, suffering – which may more productively, at some point, be redistributed across the broader matrix of the group.

It can be entirely appropriate at times for an individual's narrative to take precedence in a group. Monologuing is part of communicational diversity in groups. Unrelenting, however, it monopolises resources, breeds resentment rather than empathy and can be a form of resistance to dialogue and discourse. Some reasons for such behaviour are referred to in Chapter 4. High levels of anxiety and/or the monopoliser's conviction that they are neither heard nor understood may also prompt this form of communication (Behr and Hearst 2005). The conductor, however, needs also to consider motivations emanating from the group. For example, is the monopoliser going unchallenged because thereby the group evacuates their own greed? If so, any intervention will need to stimulate thought about what interpersonal dynamic is being (re)enacted rather than simply challenging, or even analysing, the individual or enforcing a conversational rule.

Similar motivating forces may be at work in a group that adopts turn-taking. Although perhaps appearing helpful, turn-taking quickly proves a stultifying way of interacting (or not interacting). If adopted unconsciously, an intervention bringing it to the group's attention may be enough to either make the process available for analysis or prompt diversity of opinion with regard its merits. If arrived at by more or less unanimous conscious decision, a more interpretative intervention (about the anxieties against which turn-taking might defend) may be required.

In the context, say, of a group discussion about whether group therapy really provides for individual needs, turn-taking might be understood as a 'restrictive solution' to a 'focal conflict' (Whitaker and Lieberman 1964) – for example the conflict between a desire for 'me' time ('disturbing motive') on the one hand and a fear of rejection ('reactive motive') on the other. In an effort to resolve tensions aroused by this focal conflict, a mechanistic, turn-taking model of exchange might evolve. This circumvents the problem, allowing contact to continue, though without any further exploration of the original theme. Since the manner in which groups resolve such conflicts is key to developing group culture, and since turn-taking is counter to the group analytic culture of free-floating discussion, the conductor may need to intervene to stop the restrictive solution and promote a more 'enabling' one. Enabling solutions – those which reduce anxiety but allow thematic explorations to continue – produce enabling cultures more in line with that of group analysis. Nonetheless, restrictive solutions may be necessary, at times, to reduce tensions enough to continue at all. For this reason, the conductor may refrain from intervening, waiting instead to see if the restrictive solution runs its course.

Perhaps most problematic – and certainly amongst the most challenging moments – are conversations between two sides (either individual or sub-groups) locked in confrontation. Confrontation is important. Potentially, it provides different perspectives, feeding an acknowledgement of difference. Further, it can help develop group confidence in its capacity to survive, contain and integrate aspects of competition, aggression, conflict and the expression of complex and diverse needs. However, where confrontation has a marked lack of tolerance and marked presence of contempt and/or disgust and the group, other than the 'pair', appear voyeuristic and/or paralysed, the conductor must intervene.

The manner of intervention will depend upon the maturity of the group. In a relatively new group, it may be necessary to stop the interaction with a comment such as, 'This is a very important fight. But not now.' This, of course, may well draw aggression onto the conductor. Alternatively, if the conductor has a good enough understanding of the nature of the malignant mirroring at work, a direct interpretation may be of use. More useful, if the group seems robust enough, is to invite other members to comment on *their* experience. This is to reopen the wider communicational processes in the matrix and may lead to deeper understanding not only of mutual projections between the main protagonists but of the likely projections at work in the group-as-a-whole which have become located in this specific relational conflict.

Working with resistance against being 'independent'

Dependence is an essential foundation for the development of independence. Without a cherished experience of dependence there can be no basic trust and without basic trust there can be no real intimacy. In the intimacy that is dependence we learn most deeply, and in the loss inherent in separating from that upon which we have grown dependent we make what we learn our own. Such painfully, hard-won, inner resources are what give us our so-called 'independence' or, from a group analytic perspective, our 'inter-dependence', since this reflects better the reality in which identity grows.

In a group, particularly early in its life, individual members often seek support from the conductor. For example, questions addressed directly to him are not uncommon. Sensitively frustrating these by asking what prompted them or redirecting them to the group usually quickly helps contribute to a culture of inter-dependence. However, even though careful selection may temper such dynamics, intense, primitive dependency needs can emerge at any time, either at an individual or at a group level. Such dynamics are considered more fully in Chapters 6 and 7.

Working with resistance to joining the matrix

Almost every group has its 'isolates' – 'individuals who rarely . . . make an effort to understand and attach themselves' (Ormont 2004: 65). Isolates do not have the capacity for 'transient identifications' – the ability to identify with others, without losing themselves entirely to and in others. Since those with this capacity are better able to understand, learn from, reveal to and be enriched by others (Scheidlinger 1964), drawing the isolate into the group flow becomes an essential therapeutic task. Whilst some analysts see isolation as dissolving naturally 'in the temperate mix of group communication' (Behr 2004: 76), for others, the conductor needs to be particularly active in drawing the isolate in.

Understanding communicated by some members towards group 'isolates' (either spontaneously or at the conductor's invitation) is an example of how such vital connections begin to be made. Further, invitations to isolates to contribute what they understand about another member's predicament or feeling state can also be beneficial since not only does the member in question feel understood, but the isolate experiences something of what it is to understand. However, there will be compelling reasons for an isolate's resistance to connecting with others, and unless these are understood, simple invitations to connect in understanding are unlikely to be very productive.

'The driving reason for isolation is always the disowning of a feeling ... "If I avoid others, I won't have to feel this or that way"' (Ormont 2004: 69). In Ormont's model, the conductor works both through the group and with the individual to bring these unwanted feelings (and the communicational patterns adopted to protect him from them) to the isolate's attention. The resulting conversion of isolation into loneliness can be a painfully slow one. This is particularly so when isolates, rather than experiencing their isolation as an impediment, present in 'contained guise', 'devoid of emotional colouring', bearing their relational state with 'relatively passive acceptance' and equanimity (Behr 2004: 79). Further, vital to the therapeutic process is that 'not only does the group enter the world of the isolate, but the isolate [by means of relocation and acknowledgement, by the group, of unacceptable feelings] enters the world of the group' (p. 80).[4]

Sometimes one or two group members appear to engage with the group, but in role as (co)therapist rather than equal participant. Of course, group therapy encourages members' capacity to be therapist to others. This capacity may even, appropriately at times, emerge through the offering of consciously proffered interpretations. Such offerings can be valuable not only for their content (which can be mutative for the recipient) but because they may help consolidate a growing sense of insight, authority and worth on the part of the interpreter. However, they can also be more imitative than authentic; a defence against deeper communication, perhaps rivalling the conductor, perhaps competing with siblings for special 'married' status as 'assistant conductor' (Foulkes 1975a/1986: 117), perhaps projecting vulnerability and need into those proffered their interpretative gifts. Should this be the case, an initial intervention might be one that both values the contribution *and* invites a personal response. If this fails to shift the communicational pattern, a more challenging intervention might be required. Most helpfully, this will come from the group, which is unlikely to tolerate such an approach for long.

Collective resistance to joining the matrix can be particularly destructive (Pines and Roberts 1992). Understanding its source must become a prime focus for the conductor. Although the conductor's 'feather'-like intervention can favourably tilt the process along more developmental lines (Roberts 1991), more robust interpretative interventions may be required.

Working with resisting integrating difference

Not only may those who feel isolated resist joining the group, the group may resist integrating the isolated. Such resistance may be symptomatic of a collaborative quarantine in which a disturbance in the group is not only located in an individual but, by means of projective mechanisms, locked there (see 'personification' in Chapter 3). Although an individual so identified may fit the role assigned them, the conductor needs to think in terms of not only the individual's history (their personal matrix) prompting them to take up such a position but the way in which the dynamic matrix of the group may be using the individual to avoid integration of unwanted aspects of itself.

Though there is often a psychological 'fit' on the part of a scapegoat, there is not necessarily so. An identifiable 'difference' that threatens the fantasised integrity of the group can be enough to elicit abuse. Foulkes suggests scapegoating results from displaced aggression – a group member being chosen, unconsciously, as a stand-in for the conductor. Consequently, the conductor needs to draw the aggression towards himself. Causes of scapegoating, however, are likely to be more diverse. Certainly, traumatised groups experiencing high levels of threat are particularly vulnerable to the temporary relief afforded them by this phenomenon. Conformity provides safety for the majority by demanding the eradication and/or expulsion of that which is 'bad', humiliating, shameful, different. Whatever the conductor's responding intervention, he cannot afford to remain silent for long.

When there are socially charged differences in a group – for example around ethnicity, class, disability, sexuality and gender – it is particularly important for the conductor to keep in mind not only the usual projective processes but those aspects of the social unconscious which inevitably penetrate the dynamic matrix of the group, including the conductor. Often, rather than leading to overt expressions of prejudice, repressive forces can produce a tacit agreement not to broach the taboo subject – in effect denying difference. The conductor must not shy away from challenging such unconscious 'gagging injunctions' or from foregrounding differences which otherwise might be kept secret. Once the 'secret' is out and the oppressed group members are spoken about, both the individual/sub-group concerned and the group-as-a-whole are usually better able to engage in productive discourse (Blackwell 1994; Rippa 1994). Such discourse is rarely easy, however, since we are all penetrated by the social to the core (and thus by the social unconscious) and are not only prey to its forces but often deeply ashamed of being so.

Working with silence as resistance

Silence has many meanings. It accompanies moments of deep reflection as well as of isolation and withdrawal, of communion as well as communicative resistance. If the latter, and if prolonged, the conductor must intervene.

When silence is pervasive, a simple observation of it, or enquiry about it, is often enough to reestablish connections. If it isn't, an interpretation may help. However, even if the conductor, drawing on their observations of the group and of his countertransference, feels quite confident about his interpretation, it is often preferable to deliver it half-formed (for example, as a series of observations or as a 'thought-in-progress') than fully so.

When resistant silence is located in an individual, it is more difficult for the conductor to enquire directly. Not only can doing so develop a group culture of depending on the conductor but such direct enquiries are often experienced as particularly penetrating and it is always better if other members of the group are moved to engage instead. Further, since the conductor cannot hope to attend to each individual all the time, helping the group develop its capacity to 'hold' its members is preferable to the conductor always attempting to do so. If the group appears to ignore the individual, this observation is itself worth making, prompting thought perhaps about what connections the group is wary of making. In effect, what is the individual not communicating on behalf of the group?

Working with resistance to staying

In the wake of sudden drop-out, there is little a conductor can do other than help the group process that wake. Staying alert to the premonitory signs – late-coming, irregular attendance, withdrawal from interaction – and intervening earlier is likely to be more beneficial. Even if such intervention does not prevent drop-out, it is more likely to protect the group from a sense of impotence, failure and persecutory guilt. Often, enabling the individual concerned to speak openly about their thoughts is enough to prompt resonances in the group, so helping the potential drop-out feel less isolated.[5]

Resistance to ending

In a slow open group, where patients leave gradually and hopefully with good notice, group members experience several endings during their time in the group. Since 'the failure to negotiate endings effectively is one of the key causes of intrapsychic and interpersonal difficulties' (Barnes et al. 1999: 96), such experiences offer important opportunities for reparative work.

Nevertheless, the intense, primitive feelings provoked by endings (in those who leave and those who are left) make regression common. Old symptoms/ behaviour patterns often reemerge, mourning processes come into play and the value of the group may be idealised (as if without it, nothing good will remain) as easily as it may be denigrated (as if nothing good has ever been achieved). The conductor must help the group talk and think about these recapitulations. In so doing, he may find it helpful to remember that such regressive dynamics, though transferentially and countertransferentially powerful, are usually temporary and an important part of the work (Maar 1989; Ward 1989). Of course, the group will have had plenty of rehearsals for such explorations in response to absences and breaks.

In a time-limited group, it is the conductor, not the patient, who makes the final decision about ending. It is particularly important, then, that he retains responsibility for alerting the group to the ending and encouraging the sharing of thoughts and feelings in this respect, noting aloud when the group appears resistant, verbalising, if necessary, some of the conflicted feelings that may be evoked, as well as possible concerns about the future. In effect, the conductor often becomes more active, emphasising the shared nature of the process and usually offering more group-as-a-whole observations. This tends to evoke recollection, reflection and an intensification of feedback. Some conductors actively elicit evaluations – a consideration of what has been gained as well as what has not been addressed.

Sometimes, final sessions are characterised by concrete offerings and acts of sharing. Someone brings cake, another drink, others cards, gifts. These run counter to the principle of abstinence. There is little point, however, in launching into interpretations – at least not immediately. More productive may be an initial accommodation of them before engaging in reflection. The desire to go on sharing, to give and receive, whether there will be any sustaining food once the group ends – these are some of the reflections that might be usefully encouraged in a context of social tolerance rather than analytic austerity.

Conclusion

Somewhat tongue-in-cheek, group analysis has been described as 'therapy for grown-ups'. This refers to the fact that patients must relinquish the fantasy of being made better by the parent-conductor and seek succour instead in the wider, richer matrix of group life. The conductor too must relinquish the omnipotent fantasy of providing each individual with the crucial therapeutic intervention. If such fantasies are not relinquished, both conductor and group are destined to be wedded to an impossible, ultimately dispiriting task.

The conductor builds, develops and maintains the group as both therapeutic medium and agent of change. Engaging freely in the processes of resonance, mirroring and exchange, such a group associates at all communicational levels and develops, over time, greater coherence, confidence in its authority, outsight and insight, and capacity for translation. The conductor guides such development, carefully selecting and preparing its members and managing and guarding the group's boundaries. Within the boundaries of the therapeutic frame, he takes a position that is both different from and similar to his patients', utilising his observations of self-in-interaction (including the countertransference) and others-in-interaction (including the transference) to offer a presence that 'intervenes' (holds and contains) as well as an actively intervening presence. Together, these encourage the generative momentum arising out of a creative tension between integrative and analytic forces, enabling the group to progress through constructive, deconstructive and reconstructive experiences (Schlapobersky and Pines 2009), fuelled by the increasingly complex and meaningful web of communication that is the dynamic matrix of the group. As Barnes et al. (1999) note, 'The group exists for the benefit of the individual members, yet they can only benefit by giving up aspects of themselves to the group.' And this is exactly what the conductor must do if, by dint of what he is, as well as what he does, he is to 'foster an understanding of the group as an entity that is more than the individuals' (p. 124), that is 'different from the sum of its parts' (Lewin 1951: 146).

Notes

1 Nitsun (2009) links Foulkes' aversion to directive leadership to the experience of pathological leadership figures of World War II (p. 326).
2 The table, for Foulkes, provides a focal object, reducing the empty space. It can also become a transitional object (Kosseff 1975).
3 Amongst group analytic blind spots, Prodgers (1991) suggests 'a tendency to emphasize the constructive, holding capacities of the group at the expense of its destructive, enmeshing or isolating potential' (p. 400).
4 Behr (2004) also notes those experiencing culturally determined isolation – 'a sense of not belonging which stems more from the foundation matrix . . . than from the individual's psychopathology . . . This form of isolation . . . built around racial, ethnic, religious, language or gender differences' (p. 81) requires active work on the part of the conductor in drawing attention to it and helping the group find words to explore it.
5 In response to a sudden drop-out, a conductor may offer one or more individual sessions in an effort to bridge the communicational gulf between individual and group.

Chapter 6

Developments in group analysis
The mother approach

Nick Barwick

An appreciation of the mother–infant paradigm – of how the infant mind forms in interaction with the primary care-giver (for reasons of culture and simplicity, often referred to as 'mother') – though never elaborated by Foulkes, is implicit in group analysis from the start. Referring to the 'group-as-mother', Foulkes (1948/1983) expresses an essential optimism about the group's capacity to nurture; an optimism nicely captured by Pines (1978):

> At a very deep unconscious level this group, an entity greater than any one member, on which all are dependent, which all need to be valued and accepted by, which nourishes them with its warmth, which accepts all parts of them, that understands pain and suffering, that is patient yet uncompromising, that is destroyed neither by greedy possessive primitive love, nor by destructive anger, that has permanence and continuity in time and space, this entity is basically a mother.
>
> Pines (1978: 122)

Foulkes' group analytic model challenges Freudian, one-person psychology; a psychology that construes the individual mind, dominated by innate drives, as a relatively closed system. However, as post-WWII psychoanalysis itself underwent radical change, developing along far more relational lines, the emerging two-person psychological perspective, with its appreciation, enshrined in the mother–infant paradigm, of the fundamental significance of the interaction between external and internal in the formation of intra-psychic structure, offered group analysis analytic allies with rich theoretical veins to mine.

Containing

Containing is a psychic activity linked with projective identification. The latter, initially formulated as a primitive defence in which unwanted, unmanageable aspects of self are evacuated into another (Klein 1946/1988; Bion 1962a/1984) developed to include its function as primitive form of communication. The newborn infant – no longer held within the all-providing intra-uterine environment and lacking cognitive capacities to make sense of unfamiliar, often alarming, 'raw experience' – projects the resulting psychic disturbance into mother, eliciting a mirroring anxiety within her. Ideally, out of something frightening, forever (the baby has no sense of time) and formless, mother, in 'reverie' (Bion 1970) – a relaxed condition where meaning is not made prematurely but arises out of the full, often uncomfortable evidence of experience – makes a thought: you are cold; you are hungry; you are lonely. Acting on this thought, she responds to baby's needs. Baby, in the wake of repeated attuned responses, thus experiences both *being* understood and *trust* in being understood. Building a lexicon of experience based on mother's meaningful responses, he introjects not only thoughts but the mental apparatus for thinking. Indeed, from experience, he learns that new, disorienting experiences, even when prompting disturbing anxieties[1], can be tolerated and, in the end, made sense of; that is, they can be contained. Thus, though the containing process becomes an intra-psychic activity, it is learnt through, and remains embedded in, a relational context.

Much of our experience, however, is never adequately contained. This may be because of the inadequacy of the container – a primary care-giver distracted, preoccupied, depressed, intolerant, abusive and/or rejecting – or because of the virulence of the projections. Whichever the cause(s), where containment fails, problematic feeling states remain unintegrated, aspects of 'the unthought known' (Bollas 1987). Consequently, still prey to psychic disturbance, we resort to intensified projective identifications to gain temporary relief, even if no longer hopeful of containment. All this is to recognise that the need for containment fits well Foulkes' own conviction that 'the real nature of the mind lies in each individual's need for communication and reception, in every sense of the term' (1974/1990: 278).

The therapist works to contain the as yet uncontained, projected aspects of the patient, re-presenting them in a more digestible (thoughtful) form in an effort to develop the patient's capacity to contain him/herself. In the face of patient projective identifications, the therapist 'invites invasion but resists capture' (Segal 1977). This challenging, intra- and inter-psychic work can be understood in terms of working with the countertransference (Ogden 1979).

In groups, the conductor uses countertransference to contain not only individual but sub-group and group-as-a-whole projections. The impact of this work can be considerable. Still greater complexities arise from the fact that all members and the group-as-a-whole engage in projective identification not only with the conductor but with each other. This can be a mixed blessing. Early in the formation of a group, such projections can lead to antagonism and disproportionate distrust. Alternatively, they may bring about a narcissistic 'fusion' with, and idealisation of, the group and/or conductor. Although the latter is problematic long-term, initially it can help provide necessary (and developmental) cohesion (Battegay 1994).

Projective identification offers 'endless possibilities for the open expression of denied feelings' (Rogers 1987: 100). Yet when these projections over-accumulate and petrify, they can also be immensely destructive. Scapegoating and malignant mirroring exemplify this. In scapegoating, for example, the 'sins' of the group are projected into the 'goat'/'other'. Acting on them, the 'other', with apparent justification, is then ousted/'sacrificed' for the good of the now 'cleansed' in-crowd. As a variation on this, in malignant mirroring, shameful, detested aspects of self are mutually projected into the mirror of the other, cementing a perverse psychological fit.[2]

The capacity to contain not only one's own psychic contents but those of others (at some level, essentially indivisible) is an important psychic achievement and one usefully learnt in groups. Yet the container also needs robust support attuned to the level of their containing capacity. That is to say, the container needs containing. In groups, this may necessitate speedy intervention by the conductor, if not to contain, to prevent abuse. Ultimately, however, the conductor seeks to facilitate the development of the group's containing function. To this end, the very notion of developing ever more articulate forms of communication and at ever deeper levels – that is, 'putting it into words' – becomes a form of containment; containment that helps develop the group's faith in its capacity to contain (see Zinkin 1989).

We are all projectors and containers. Even mothers, especially when poorly contained, project aspects of themselves, be they idealised, denigrated, feared or longed for, into their infants. The conductor thus needs to be alert to his own potential (ab)use of the group. Although training and personal analysis should minimise such intrusions, they are also inevitable. What makes the difference is how self-reflection, supported by supervision and other containing relationships, help the conductor work creatively with such containment 'failures'. To acknowledge this intersubjectivity gives new meaning to Foulkes' (1964) comment that the conductor's personality has an 'overwhelming influence' on the group.

Holding, surviving, playing

'Holding' describes mother's attuned response to infant need. Such dependability implies mother's love and it is within this 'total environmental provision' (Winnicott 1960/1990) that the infant, largely protected from the grosser impingements of reality (and of accompanying anxieties) develops a growing sense of 'continuity of being'. In effect, mother acts as baby's 'auxiliary ego' while baby, relatively unperturbed, is left to discover its primitive, coherent, authentic identity/'True Self'.

As the infant self coheres, the holding environment loosens. Emerging from a state of attuned 'madness' called 'primary maternal preoccupation' (Winnicott 1956/1992), mother begins to rediscover her own (separate) mind and the infant begins to experience the 'impingement' of small 'doses of reality'. Not everything happens when he wants it; between a need and a satisfaction, a gap appears.

Gaps resulting from brief, well-timed impingements help the infant gain a sense of separateness and develop psychic muscle. However, impingements that are too early or too intense provoke not the experience of a loosening hold but of being 'let down', 'dropped', forever 'falling'. Defending against such 'drops', the infant reactively holds himself. The formation of a 'False/Caretaker Self' is just such a 'reactive' self-holding.

Developing psychic muscle, he tests out his environment to see if it can withstand his growing strength. Only when he discovers that the 'object mother' – the mother who, in the primitive infant mind, being distinct from the caring 'environmental mother', is the one against whom he directs his aggression – can 'survive', can he be confident of his own separateness and begin to develop concern for the other (Winnicott 1963/1990). Indeed, through the non-retaliatory, boundary-enforcing survival of the object, he finds not only confirmation of the mother's loving resilience but 'proof of [her] . . . ability to hate objectively' (Winnicott 1947/1992: 199) – that is, to hate his relentless, 'ruthless' demands and still 'hold on'. Only then, when he is wholly known, can he begin to believe in being wholly loved.

Although recognition of separateness makes available the riches of relatedness, it is not an easy transition to make. To help, the baby develops a 'transitional space'. This space arises out of the infant's creation/use of a 'transitional object' (Winnicott 1971/1974); objects imbued with 'good-mother stuff' (Deri 1978: 52). For example, a bit of blanket may seamlessly become, through sensual links with breast, infant's tongue and sucked thumb alongside which it slips, almost an extension of him (and his fantasised unity with mother/breast) and yet is not him/mother/breast. This 'intermediate area of experience' (Winnicott 1951/1992) – of a 'world' neither entirely inner, wholly subjective and omnipotently ruled, nor entirely outer, wholly objective, impotently inhabited, offers both consolation and challenge and is, for Winnicott, where imagination begins; the 'as if' of play.

Play is a resource not only for infants managing the tricky, conflicting demands of internal and external (shared) realities, but one to which we all must return, at times, as we try to negotiate, creatively, the demands of reality (its separations, losses and frustrations) without undue loss of spontaneity, of 'continuity of being'. Play allows a temporary 'withdrawal' from the full demanding force of external reality; a space in which to renew and reinvigorate connections with the 'True Self' in the service of creative living.

The capacity to play is thus a developmental achievement. Further, it is a precondition for therapeutic work which takes place in the 'overlap of two areas of playing, that of the patient and that of the therapist' (Winnicott 1971/1974: 44). If patients cannot play or cannot engage in play, therapy's first task is to ensure they can. This requires addressing the developmental need for the holding of both an empathically attuned 'environmental mother' and the availability of an exciting, frustrating, challenging 'object' one.

The analytic setting provides the holding environment which, in individual therapy, the therapist communicates by being preoccupied with the patient and placing himself at his service, being reliably present, expressing love through interest and (by keeping boundaries) expressing hate, making an effort to understand, refraining from imposing his own needs/agenda, not being hurt by fantasies, not retaliating and surviving (Winnicott 1954/1992). In a group context, such holding is communicated first by the conductor, then by the group.

Drawing on James (1984; 1994), Nitsun (1989) highlights parallels between early infant–mother relations and early group formation. The 'infant-group' inhabits a relatively unintegrated state: individuals without a sense of connectedness, continuity, cohesion. This stimulates 'archaic' anxieties about physical and psychic survival. Attuned, the conductor adopts the role of auxiliary ego, of holding environmental mother whose empathic responsiveness protects both individuals and group-as-a-whole from gross impingements and whose very presence must speak of 'reliability taken for granted' (Winnicott 1965/1989). Without such holding, anxieties may feel intolerable and early drop-out, precipitous 'False Self' formation (for example, rigid, rule-bound, self-holding which keeps the group together at the expense of spontaneity) or even group disintegration may ensue. Nitsun (1989) recommends the conductor be present 'in a tangible way to help the group feel safe, to define boundary issues clearly' rather than maintaining 'a position of determined therapeutic detachment' (p. 253)[3]. Careful attention to dynamic administration thus helps provide holding sufficient for the group to begin to cohere.

Even in a relatively coherent group, the import of holding should not be underestimated. Untoward events can provoke archaic anxieties at any time. Further, as Yogev (2008) notes, patient improvement often comes as much through 'the expansion' as 'the challenging of the emotional space' and it is exactly such expansion – of the capacity to be and be with – in an environment suitably protected from 'aversive stimuli from his surroundings' (p. 376), that holding in a group provides.

In group analytic groups, holding is a mutual activity with multiple axes. Although modelled by the conductor, each member finds him/herself in a position of holding as well as of being held. The individual's and group-as-a-whole's growing capacities to hold others is indicative of psychological maturity.

A quality necessary for holding others is the capacity to withhold oneself; holding back (though never losing touch with) one's own subjective experience in the service of meeting another's needs, even when those needs include what can be quite aggressive explorations. Paradoxically, such withholding promotes individual expansion. This is so, not only because it strengthens self-efficacy but also because it helps develop the capacity to tolerate difference, that essential ingredient in the development of identity. Further, the group that manages to hold, withhold and 'hold on' (that is, survive without retaliating) in the face of turbulent elaborations of identity – aggression being an integral part of appetite, motility and creativity (Winnicott 1964/1991) – helps allay fears of relational catastrophe in the face of such turbulence and develops the group's confidence in, and capacity to, play.[4]

Winnicott played a game with young patients called the 'squiggle game' (1968/1989). The child drew something, then Winnicott added something of his own. This to and fro 'communication' continued until something emerged that was satisfying and recognisable to the child, though it was a shared creation, coming into being within a transitional space. This describes well an analytic group at play: multiple, interacting squiggles (free discussion) from which both highly personalised and shared meanings arise within a uniquely personalised yet shared space. Co-created language with frequent references to aspects of group history and myth and the elaborate construction and use of co-created metaphor is often characteristic of such play. Such play loosens, frees, since play does not have real implications; it does not, for example, destroy, since what is played with is not real, even if the feelings evoked are real. All this can lead to a great deal of experimentation in the service of living (Jacobson 1989).

Within the 'mutual sphere of creative illusion' created by a therapy group, 'gently, and little by little, the group helps the individual to alter his subjective perception of reality as his individual transitional space becomes more interactive with the group space' (Schlachet 1986: 47). This shared, overlapping experience of play, a patient tellingly describes:

> It is all, it is nothing.
>   It is real, it is pretend.
>   Family – father, mothers, sisters, brothers, they are all here, yet they are not.
>   Lovers, friends, husbands, wives, companions, enemies, they are all here, yet they are not.
>   Joy, pain, love, hate, understanding, confusion, communication, conflict, they are all here and they are not.
>   . . . .
>   And so, we will all, in our way, profit by it, learn from it, live better from it.
>   Because, you see, it is painful, but it is not.
>
> Schlachet (1986: 51)

A secure base

Bowlby's work on 'attachment' (1979) and the 'secure base' (1988) has had a significant influence on the theory and practice of therapy and group analysis is no exception (Marrone 1994; 1998). Developments in understanding affect regulation and mentalisation (how we make and use mental representations of our own and other people's emotional states) are amongst the advances in developmental theory informed by attachment theory (Fonagy et al. 2002) and these too have begun to be considered by group analysis, particularly when working with patients with severely disorganised attachments (Karterud 2011). It is not my intention, however, to elaborate any such aspects here since these are explored in Chapters 9 and 10.

Empathising

Empathy has long been significant in therapeutic encounter. Over the last few decades, however, its significance has grown from contributing factor in the therapeutic alliance, to research tool in understanding the patient's internal world to, particularly through self-psychology and its offspring, intersubjectivity, a role equal to, if not greater than, interpretation in eliciting psychological transformation.

Empathy's raised significance arises out of recognition of its fundamental contribution to the development of self. From a self-psychological perspective, 'empathic resonance' (Kohut 1977) – dependent upon parental capacity to empathise with the child – provides the medium in which narcissistic needs (referred to as selfobject needs since they relate to various experiences of merger with the object) can be satisfactorily met. These needs – to be mirrored (in the gaze of the parents), to idealise (the parent imago: 'You are perfect; but then, I'm part of you' (Kohut 1971: 27)) and for twinship – if met, proffer, respectively, a sense of self-worth, purpose/self-control and belonging. (Later, Wolf (1988) adds adversarial need: the need to engage with a benign adversary in order to test and develop strength and enjoy healthy competition.)

Just as empathic resonance allows robust development of self, organised around satisfying selfobject experiences, self-psychology identifies its absence as the root cause of most psychological disturbance. Without an ambience of empathy, unmet needs leave the relatively incohesive self floundering in chaotic, narcissistic immaturity, desperately seeking relational contexts which might provide what is lacking and/or, fearing further traumatising disappointment, avoiding relational connection altogether.

Although unmet narcissistic needs are traumatising, given a foundation of adequate selfobject experiences, the self's maturation is furthered by conditions of 'optimal failures' since 'tolerable disappointments . . . lead to the establishment of internal structures which provide the basis for self-soothing' (Kohut 1984: 64). It is the creative use of empathic failure within a field of mostly sustained empathic resonance that gives therapy its momentum (Chused and Raphling 1992).

Empathically born selfobject experiences are readily available in group analytic groups. Under the '"me-in-you, you-in-me" rhythm', experience of mirroring helps develop self-worth. Further, as group cohesiveness develops, the group comes to represent a 'powerful, calming resource' (Roberts and Pines 1992: 476) – an idealised selfobject – with comments such as 'I can relate to that' articulating the meeting of twinship needs. Lastly, adversarial needs may be more readily met in a group than in a dyad, owing to greater diversity in power relations and consequent increased freedom/safety to experiment.

Contemporary infant research shows infants, from the earliest weeks, engaging in 'evocative behaviour' designed to obtain empathic responses necessary for development. An infant whose environment includes extended family may thus have 'a greater probability of obtaining the responsiveness and the selfobject functions it requires'. Indeed, several consistent selfobjects may 'enhance the diversity of the symbolic structure [of self] being organised' (Harwood 1986: 293–4). This is particularly important if the primary caretaker is disturbed since availability of alternative intersubjective matrices helps supplement otherwise restricted mental repertoires for living. Potentially, a group offers just such a bolstering diversity of selfobject experience.

With the maturation of self comes recognition of 'the relatively independent center of initiative in the other' (Ornstein 1981: 358). Individuals aware of both self and other in this way are able to engage in 'reciprocal empathic resonance' (Wolf 1980), leading to greater availability of satisfactory selfobject experiences. Indeed, 'one of the therapist's most important functions will be to facilitate reciprocal empathic resonance as a coordinate of the spontaneous reactiveness that comprises the vitality of the therapeutic group' (Bacal 1985a: 499; see also 1991; 1998).

The conductor promotes empathic resonance by adopting an attitude of 'optimal responsiveness' (Bacal 1985b) – a view in line with contemporary infant research into the nature of the relational environments best suited to psychological development. Indeed, exploring 'non-interpretive mechanisms' in therapy, Stern et al. (1998) refer to those 'special moments' of 'authentic person-to-person connection' or 'moments of meeting' involving 'implicit relational knowing' and complex 'affect attunement' that are as mutative as any interpretation. In group analysis, such moments are not limited to those between group member and conductor. However, the conductor's empathy can significantly promote a milieu of empathic reciprocity characteristic of a mature group.

Drawing on neuroscientific and psychological studies, Nava (2007) speculates on the nature of empathy at work in the analytic process. Focusing mainly upon the conductor's response to the patient, she suggests patients' emotions 'are mirrored through the mirror neuron [see Chapter 4] in the neuronal circuits that codify the same emotion in the analyst' (Nava 2007: 20). Such affect-sharing, achieved naturally if not defended against, is communicated through the mirroring of affect in our faces. Affect-sharing, however, can cause 'emotional contagion' (Preston and de Waal 2002: 6) – a type of merger between empathising subject and object empathised with. This prevents the former maintaining sufficient separateness to be able to offer help. Thus the conductor utilises training, supervision and personal analysis to 'resist capture'. Lastly, mental flexibility and auto-regulation come into play. These involve using personal knowledge, beliefs and experience (in other words, 'self-perspective') to step into the other's shoes whilst, at the same time, regulating/inhibiting that very same self-perspective.

Where, in the group, defences against affect-sharing are evident, where emotional contagion threatens to consume, or where forms of colonisation of the other (because self-perspective is not sufficiently regulated) dominate, the conductor will need to draw the group's attention. Helpful will be the conductor's own capacity to maintain fairly sophisticated levels of empathic engagement and, when not able to, to reflect upon, be open to and even prompt discussion about, empathic failure. For group members, observing and imagining this is likely, by means of mirror neurons (Rizzolatti et al. 2001), to lead to significant learning – a type of 'empathy training-in-action'. The 'curriculum objectives' of such training might be to develop empathic ability along three continuums (Yogev 2013):

- The resonance continuum: the ability to observe and recognise (often unconscious) emotional information transmitted
- The comprehension continuum: the ability to determine what belongs to oneself and what belongs to others
- The identification of needs continuum: the ability to prioritise between needs both within oneself and in relation to others

and two dimensions:

- The non-verbal/facial
- The verbal

A group offers ample opportunity to observe empathic sensitivity, addressing 'developmental deficiencies in empathy' (Yogev 2013: 73) where necessary. Further, the effect of such empathy-training is to help establish a group culture in which new members, perhaps less empathically developed, can learn from the normative interpersonal and intersubjective interactions of the group according to principles of 'perception-action liaison' (Prinz 1997).

To acknowledge both being empathic and being empathised with as core aspects of development is to appreciate the deep, mutually creative, intersubjective nature of the mother–infant paradigm. For the mother who bears a child with whom, empathising, she feels compassion (the latter being 'an expansion of the capacity for empathy' (Segalla 2012: 137)) is herself re-born within the mother–infant, intersubjective field. To put it another way, 'finding the other through empathy and compassion is the way to find the self' (p. 136).

Along these lines, philosophers Buber, Gadamer and Levinas all conclude, suggests Orange (2009 cited in Segalla 2012), that concepts of individuality have served us badly over the years and 'so invite us to develop a therapeutic culture in which generosity, care and protection of the other become our central values' (p. 11). After all, as Gadamer notes, 'It is the other who breaks my self-centredness [and so my prison] by giving me something to understand' (p. 148).

The 'other' mother

Foulkes emphasises the group as 'all embracing mother'. Prodgers (1990) suggests this neglects the negative transference to the 'group-as-a-whole'; transference based on subjective *and* objective experiences of frightening and/or deficient mothering. Denial of this essential ambivalence may be necessary initially in a group, counteracting mistrust that would otherwise inhibit cohesive forces vital to collaboration. Long-term, however, it leads to splitting; an idealised group-mother and denigrated/feared conductor, for example, or 'castrated' group-mother and powerful, protective conductor-father (Gibbard and Hartman 1973; Raphael-Leff 1984).

Drawing on analytical psychology (Neumann 1963), Prodgers (1990) elaborates the notion of the feminine, differentiating 'elementary' and 'transformational' characteristics, each of which has positive and negative aspects. An elementary characteristic of the mother is the 'Great Round': the vessel/group that 'contains and holds fast onto everything within it' (p. 22); protecting, sheltering. Yet that which it contains is dependent upon it; 'utterly at its mercy'. Such a mother may, therefore, also restrict, ensnare, devour. In contrast, the transformative mother is characterised by movement. Again, however, she is two-sided. Symbolised as bearing and releasing seeds from the pod, she encourages change, development, individuation as well as abandons, deprives, rejects.

The experience of the negative mother (in both elementary and transformative guises) appears particularly prominent in larger groups. However, though less foregrounded, she may still be evident in smaller ones:

> The most intense group-induced anxiety – recapitulating early developmental sequences of psychological differentiation – is the annihilation of self, either through engulfment and fusion with collectivity at one extreme, or through isolation from abandonment by the group at the other.
>
> Green (1983: 4)

Prodgers (1990) suggests Foulkes' (and most subsequent group analysts') idealisation of the mother is a professional 'blind spot' rooted in a relationship to mother inherited perhaps from Foulkes or indeed from Freud (see Rycroft 1985). Prodgers offers not only a Jungian-influenced redress but a Bionian one and it is to Bion's work, and group analysis's relationship with it, that we now turn.

Notes

1 Any new experience of which it is not yet possible to make sense evokes anxiety because it re-awakens a primitive sense of absence. This resonates with early experiences of absence of the good, nurturing breast. The good breast's absence not only prompts understandable survival anxieties but, according to Kleinian thinking, leaves us in the presence of the bad breast, a depository of all our hatred and aggression. The capacity to bear a state of 'not knowing' characteristic of absence, change and loss, thus demands considerable psychic resilience. Bion referred to this resilience, a prerequisite for creativity, as 'negative capability': the capacity to dwell in 'uncertainties, mysteries, doubts, without any irritable reaching after fact and reason' (Keats cited in Bion 1970: 125).
2 Indeed, the group itself may be projecting into the protagonist's psychic aspects which it feels unable to resolve or hold together.
3 I am reminded of Guntrip's recollection of a session with Winnicott where, having spent some time exploring Guntrip's experience of an early mother who failed to relate,

Winnicott said, 'I've nothing particular to say yet, but if I don't say something, you may begin to feel I'm not here' (Guntrip 1975 cited in Symington 1986: 308).
4 Ashbach and Schermer (1987), drawing on James (1982), describe the therapy group itself as a transitional object. First, the group gradually replaces the therapist as a source of succour and security. Second, though imagined into being, it is also a pre-existent reality. Third, 'under the proper circumstances it allows the membership to develop their cultural potential' – to play (p. 61).

Chapter 7

Developments in group analysis
The 'other'[1] approach

Nick Barwick

Bion's basic assumptions

For Bion, as for Foulkes, 'the group is essential to the fulfilment of a man's mental life' (Bion 1961: 53). Unlike Foulkes, for Bion, this inseparability is fundamentally problematic:

> The individual is a group animal at war, not simply with the group, but with himself for being a group animal and with those aspects of his personality that constitute his groupishness.
>
> Bion (1961: 131)

In response to such conflict, argues Bion, the group deploys collaborative defences. These defences undermine the group's capacity to think, to function as a 'work group' (W), cultivating instead a primitive 'group mentality' that manifests itself in the form of basic assumptions (ba) – shared, unconscious beliefs about a group's function/purpose, characterised by shared behaviour. Bion identifies three such assumptions.

Basic assumption dependency (baD)

In baD, the assumption is the group meets to make the group feel safe. To this end, it invests omnipotent and omniscient qualities in its leader. In such a dependency 'culture', where a timeless quality allays separation-anxiety, the remaining membership becomes de-skilled. Sometimes, particular members become identified as especially inadequate and in need of care.

Basic assumption fight-flight (baF)

In baF, the group meets to preserve itself. This is done by fighting the enemy – an idea or person(s) usually identified as being outside the group – or flight. Profoundly anti-intellectual, all introspective behaviour is eschewed lest awareness of internal differences (within self and/or group) leads to conflict and feared destruction. Any member challenging this culture is vulnerable to attack. This includes the leader, whose role is to identify dangers and lead the charge/flight. A leader refusing this role may be replaced by one more responsive to the group's paranoid demands.

Basic assumption pairing (baP)

In baP, the group invests hope in two or more people 'getting together' and coming up with the 'solution'. In this way, the rest of the group protects itself from anxieties related to thinking and working. In particular, it protects itself from change (with all its potential losses, conflicts and catastrophes), since what is achieved is hope of a solution rather than the solution itself. Indeed, a pair/working party that proffers a solution is rarely welcomed. Thus Bion refers to baP hope as 'Messianic'; hope that 'must never be fulfilled' since, 'Only by remaining a hope does hope persist' (1961: 151–152).

Bion versus Foulkes

Bion's essentially pessimistic, Thanatos-driven group (Schermer 1985/2000) contrasts strikingly with Foulkes's essentially optimistic, Eros-driven one. For Bion, in the face of group regressive pull, the individual's capacity to contribute creatively is severely limited. Group pressure provokes individual 'valency' – a person's propensity for picking up and acting out particular types of projections (for example aggression or dependency) and thus their 'readiness to enter into combination with another in making and acting on the basic assumptions' (Bion 1961: 116). Thus he soon becomes 'trapped, and has a fight on his hands to achieve being an individual' (Hinshelwood 2007: 349). Indeed, the only individual with a fighting chance of springing the trap is the group 'leader'. Offering group-as-a-whole interpretations, the therapist/leader strives to make conscious the forces preventing learning and change, enabling members to better manage their 'disharmonious experience of being group animals' (p. 353).

Bion's approach, elaborated by Ezriel (1973), became known as 'the Tavistock model'. Highly 'group-centred', it is a powerful way of understanding primitive processes at work in groups. However, as a therapeutic approach, outcome studies (Malan et al. 1976) revealed high levels of patient dissatisfaction, especially concerning perceived 'therapist detachment' – a seeming lack of interest in individuals which many patients found (re-)traumatising. This study helped prompt modifications (for example, Horwitz's 'inductive approach' (Horwitz 1977)). Being more sensitive to individual needs, such modifications provoke fewer anti-therapeutic reactions. However, the creative power for initiating change remains in the therapist/leader rather than the group. Given the basic premise upon which even modified 'Tavistock' approaches are built – a view of 'group mentality' wedded to Thanatos – this is not surprising.

Deeply rooted differences between Tavistock and group analytic models thus make integration difficult, though significant steps towards integration have been made nonetheless.

Behind Bion's basic assumptions

Brown (1985/2000) suggests ba phenomena are common in hierarchically structured groups. The Tavistock model, with its locus of power in the 'sphinx-like' leader, is just such a group. In contrast, in a group analytic group the conductor encourages 'spontaneous interaction and communication at many levels' – i.e. not just at the level of projection – and offers a 'flexible attitude which conveys ... a democratic spirit' (p. 210). Indeed, the conductor's interpretative restraint, coupled with efforts to transfer expert authority to the group, helps promote 'mutuality and joint endeavour' rather than hierarchy. This promotes a culture less prone to ba activity.

Nevertheless, basic assumption theory, suggests Brown, has much to offer group analysis. Since all basic assumptions may be expressions of, or reactions against, some primary state 'springing from an extremely early and primitive primal scene' (Bion 1961: 164) – that is, the child's traumatising real or fantasised witnessing of parental intercourse – Brown (1985/2000) notes that such a scene is the 'archetypal provoker of feelings of exclusion'. Hence, 'if the reality of belonging to a group does involve facing up to jealousy, envy and the frustration of dyadic dependency, it is not surprising that primitive fantasies and anxieties of this type are stirred up in an analytic group' (p. 201).

By relating ba activity to the dynamics of exclusion, Brown offers a less Thanatos-driven take on ba states. BaD is reframed as regression into mother–child merger as a defence against frustration and loss arising from the presence of others; baF becomes a way of denying rivalries for the good object by mass(ive) projection of aggression on/into objects outside the group; and baP idealises longed-for coupling whilst, because of its forever-in-the-future nature, protecting the self from envious feelings and the idealised object from envious attack. Such relational re-framing allows the conductor, faced with ba activity, to focus less on group-as-a-whole interpretations of primitive defences and more on encouraging communication about relational struggles.

In classical psychoanalysis, the primal scene is a precursor of the Oedipus Complex. Indeed, a post-Kleinian take sees both Oedipus Complex and primal scene as part of a broader 'Oedipal situation'. The infant/child is confronted with the reality of loss – of the loved object's undivided attention. The question then becomes, 'Will our love survive knowledge?' (Britton 1985/1992: 45). If we trust it will, we can look, with hope, towards the shared social world. If our doubt is greater, however, we are likely to take refuge in the 'cultivation of illusions': a retreat into the neuroses of individualism, predicated as it is on a hallucinatory capacity to satisfy self.

Nitsun (1994) considers the 'primal scene' to be 'metaphorically, humanly ... at the centre of the group' (p. 129). For example, when, following one-to-one assessments, a group begins, all members face the reality of sharing. Such sharing, echoing the loss of exclusive possession of the loved object, may re-evoke attendant anxieties, including paranoid fears of annihilation. Similar anxieties/ fears re-emerge throughout the group's life. For example, each new member/baby born out of the therapist's coupling with that which is outside the group may re-evoke them. As Foulkes suggests, 'Coping with the arrival of an infant activates regression on the part of all family members' (Foulkes 1972/1990: 238). Hence the group may experience both the threat inherent in such events *and* the opportunity to work through unresolved issues within the transference situation. Further, because the group may be unconsciously associated with the mother's body (a view with which both Foulkes and Bion concur), the very process of enquiry into the group's dynamic activity may stir anxieties related to the primal scene – the paranoid-schizoid fear of discovering part of father inside mother (a reference to the terrifying combined parent figure (Klein 1929/1988)) with its associations of retaliatory attack.

Drawing on an object relations understanding of Oedipal configurations in this way deepens the group analytic understanding of the intra-psychic drama played out in groups. Yet such drama is existential and social too; existential in that it embodies essential human notions of belonging and longing, inclusion and exclusion, the hope of creativity and the painfulness of loss; social because it deals with our efforts to come to terms with the nature of group/social processes, the developmental differentiating sequence of which group analytic therapy seeks to promote: that is, from 'self' to 'self-and-other' to 'other-and-other' to 'group'.

Beyond Bion's basic assumptions

Following Bion, three other basic assumptions have been posited:

- *Oneness* (baO) – where individuals 'surrender self for passive participation . . . lost in oceanic feelings of unity' (Turquet 1974: 357–60)
- *Me-ness* (baM) – 'a culture of selfishness in which individuals appear to be only conscious of their own personal boundaries, which they believe have to be protected from any incursion by others' (Lawrence et al. 1996: 100)
- *Incohesion: Aggregation/Massification* ((ba)I:A/M) (Hopper 1997) (see below)

The first two are from the Tavistock stable, the latter from group analysis. Our focus, then, is on the latter. However, BaM has been of particular interest to group analysis and warrants brief mention first.

Basic assumption me-ness (BaM)

BaM – referred to by Lavie (2007) as a 'group analytic basic assumption' – is a socio-culturally specific form of group mentality arising out of a crisis of faith in the reliability of the big, hitherto containing structures/institutions of state and religion. In baM, a state of 'socially induced schizoid withdrawal' (Lawrence 1996/2000: 99) where the only thing trusted is the self, the emergence of group identity is feared, threatening as it does the defensive sanctuary of individualism. Consequently, 'groupishness' is denied, shared issues being replaced by private matters and emotional engagement – dangerous because who knows what interdependence might result – by detached objectivity: 'If I were angry I would say X'. This type of exchange, Lawrence refers to as presenting a 'photograph' rather than speaking from experience. Group culture 'is ordered, calm, polite, and androgynous' (p. 110). It is also futile.

Basic assumption incohesion: Aggregation/massification ((Ba)I:A/M)

(Ba)I:A/M (Hopper 1997) combines characteristics of baO and baM in an oscillating configuration[2] but with an underpinning model of mind derived from the Independent rather than Kleinian tradition. Here, envy (and the forces of Thanatos), rather than being primary are re-framed as defensive derivatives of the virtually universal human experience of helplessness provoked by interpersonal environments that fail to provide adequate security and developmental succour. In short, (ba)I:A/M describes a group state arising out of shared traumatising experiences that have, at their centre, fears of annihilation, of falling apart, of fatal 'incohesion'. Such fears arise out of the experience either of absence of holding/containing contact or of highly invasive/engulfing contact. Both experiences threaten identity's roots, giving rise to 'contact-shunning' (where the experience has been invasive) or 'merger-hungry' (where the experience has been abandoning) behaviours.

A group's contact-shunning behaviour Hopper calls 'aggregation': 'a collection of people who have absolutely no consciousness of themselves as being members of a particular social system' (2009: 220). Characterised by 'too much individuality', the group may fall into uncommunicative silence, failing even to engage each other's gaze. In contrast, 'merger-hungry' behaviour, Hopper calls 'massification': cohesion achieved through lack of differentiation; a pseudo-cooperation or 'pulling together' motivated by inability to endure difference rather than commitment to creative connection.

Oscillation between the two states occurs because both aggregation and massification, though providing temporary relief from fear of annihilating incohesion, also give rise to it. Thus, though individuals experience identity protected when the group functions as an aggregate, they also experience threats of annihilation rooted in trauma of abandonment and/or neglect.

In (ba)I:A/M, some group members may adopt certain roles. For example, the 'lone wolf' (typical of aggregation) is adopted by those with crustacean (contact-shunning) character structures. Such members 'personify' aggregation processes, just as those with amoeboid (merger-hungry) structures may personify massification processes by adopting roles such as 'cheerleader'. Both roles draw on group aggression: the lone wolf manifesting this in cold, over-contained behaviour; the cheerleader through attacks on that which is 'other', calling for 'fatal purification of that which is different'. For this reason, 'The personification of this basic assumption must not only be met with containment and holding forever, but also subjected to understanding and interpretation' (p. 227).

In the context of the Bionian tendency to interpret and the Foulkesian tendency to 'hold', this exhortation reflects Hopper's efforts to integrate at the level of theory *and* technique.

The anti-group

The anti-group is a group analytic construct encapsulating all 'destructive processes that threaten the functioning of the group' (Nitsun 1996: 1). Heavily informed by object relations theory, in particular basic assumptions and the concept of container-contained, it is a construct intended to counter-balance Foulkes's 'excessive optimism' (Brown 2003). A product of multiple, toxic, uncontained projections provoked by the universal, conflicted experience and concomitant anxieties around belonging – the fact that the individual is a 'group animal at war' (Bion 1961) – it is an expression of Bion's group mentality. Basic assumptions, being a product of such mentality, are thus seen as specific forms of anti-group resulting from a failure of containment:

> Through projective identification, the failed group becomes impregnated with chaotic and persecutory elements of the uncontained, leaving the membership floundering in a morass of unprocessed and unresolved experience.
> Nitsun (1996: 66)

Indeed, suggests Nitsun, basic assumption groups do not really function as groups since coherent intra-group relatedness is absent. Rather, primitive, illusory dyadic relationships prevail; ones that are 'linear' (characterised by reaction and projection) rather than 'spatial' (characterised by reflection and integration) (Barwick 2004). In baD, the undifferentiated group mass looks to its leader; in baF, it looks away from (or against) its enemy; in baP, gripped by bemused and/or expectant paralysis, it looks on.

In drawing on Bion, Nitsun does not, however, turn away from Foulkes. For example, in contrast to the Bionian emphasis on group-as-a-whole interventions, Nitsun advocates addressing all levels of the interactive system: individual, subgroup and group-as-a-whole. Further, whilst Bion's approach emphasises the 'unending cycle of regression and destructiveness' (Nitsun 1996: 68), Nitsun, though noting these potentialities, emphasises the opportunities successful anti-group containment presents for mobilising group creative processes.

In considering how to 'successfully handle' the anti-group, Nitsun considers two forms of anti-group manifestation – pathological and developmental – and re-visits the conductor's influence upon these.

Handling the pathological anti-group

Nitsun cautions selecting members likely to contribute to pathological anti-group developments. For example, contra-indicated are highly aggressive individuals, particularly within a borderline personality constellation, and isolated, schizoid individuals who, in repressing rage and envy, may inhibit expression of these feelings in the group. Such inhibition encourages the anti-group to fester rather than find containment in articulation. Nevertheless, Nitsun recommends assessment according to principles of 'group membership and commitment' rather than conventional diagnostic and personality categories. Of particular relevance here are:

- *bonding capacity*, for which Adult Attachment Interviews (George et al. 1985) provide a useful assessment instrument
- *passion for proximity* (Mendez et al. 1988) as opposed to 'aversion to proximity' in interpersonal situations
- *group–object relations* – Nitsun's (1996) own term describing how individuals perceive and relate to groups.

The conductor's capacity to handle anti-group manifestations depends greatly upon his attitude to the anti-group. For example, a conductor unattuned to negative group processes is likely to prompt repression rather than expression of them, leading to potentially more insidious, pathological anti-group activity. Linked to a conductor's capacity to attune will be his attitude towards aggression. Is it seen as potentially creative or simply destructive? Such attitudes are rooted in both personal history and theoretical stance.

Acknowledging contradictions, limitations and complexities inherent in groups[3] helps members *reflect on* rather than *react to* them. 'Maintaining the group position' (Nitsun 1996: 176) – that is, resisting the anti-group tendency to focus simply on individuals – is also crucial. So too, given the anti-group's propensity for 'attacks on linking' (Bion 1959/1984) – a fragmenting, defensive mental activity that splinters connections between thought and feeling and between people – is the conductor's capacity to maintain his own 'linking function' (see Gordon 1994; Hinshelwood 1994).

Making meaningful connections is, essentially, an interpretative activity. Distinguishing between the conductor's 'broadly interpretative function' (e.g. making connections between non-conscious aspects of group communication) and 'focused interpretation' (addressing unconscious phenomena related to deeply rooted anxiety-defence constellations), Nitsun (1996) notes the former is widely valued in group analysis; the latter, less so. However, in the context of the anti-group, traditional interpretative reticence needs modifying since 'sensitively judged' focused interpretations congruent with the language, themes and metaphors of the group can ameliorate anti-group forces. Addressing individuals, prior to offering group-as-a-whole interpretations of underlying traumas prompting the anti-group, is an aspect of such 'sensitivity'. This approach can be deeply resonant and have a 'groupifying' effect (Anthony 1983).

Overall, in the face of the anti-group, especially when latent challenges to and conflicts with authority appear present, the conductor needs to take a robust, interpretative stance in order to bring these dynamics to light before they erupt into the manifest level in ways that 'derail the group and leave the members and the conductor, reeling' (Nitsun 2009: 329). Even so, Nitsun strikes a cautionary note:

> The anti-group is a sign that the therapeutic alliance in the group, often in relation to the conductor, has broken down, and with it, the capacity for reflection and insight. Making an interpretation in this context ... may therefore be counterproductive, fuelling rather than assuaging some of the primitive forces that generate the anti-group.
>
> Nitsun (1996: 180)

The anti-group, being characterised by an accumulation of aggressive responses springing from a variety of sources, requires the conductor to work towards a deconstruction of such 'defensive agglomerations'. Utilising the concept of 'location' helps trace aggression's concealed sources, making them more available to communicative process. Understanding aggression in terms of the developmental stage of the group (Gans 1989) – for example, the aggressive response that results from 'stranger anxiety' in the early part of a group or when new members join as opposed to aggression related to the struggle for control characteristic of a later stage – can also be helpful in working out how to draw hostile feelings into the communicative process. So too can an appreciation of how aggression defends against anxiety, or against the vulnerability experienced in the face of loss or intimacy or against the painful frustration of relationship needs (Rosenthal 1987). Often, to bring aggression within the field of communication, the conductor usefully draws it towards himself. This can provide a useful containing and modelling experience for the group (Tuttman 1994).

The anti-group is an 'autistic' aspect of the group, saturating primitive levels of communication. The conductor relies heavily, therefore, on his countertransference when working with it; that is, he must be sensitive to and containing of the resonances evoked and provoked in him. Although this containing capacity is, in ordinary group development, a function of the group, when the anti-group dominates, it is the function of the conductor. However, the anti-group also challenges a conductor's capacity to contain, in part because he is likely to identify himself with the group – it is his baby – and narcissistic over-identification can, in the wake of anti-group fragmentation, provoke devastating loss of confidence in both himself and the group.

Handling the developmental anti-group

The anti-group may also be construed as developmental phenomenon. For example, certain individuals/sub-groups may adopt a contrary position that aggravates the rest of the group. To re-frame such anti-group activity as projections of the group-as-a-whole and to encourage acknowledgement and integration of them can be an important developmental step. Indeed, the capacity to 'survive' the anti-group may itself be transformational. Not only does it lead to a more realistic evaluation of destructiveness (i.e. aggression is containable and not necessarily catastrophe-inducing), it may also lead to shared responsibility for the group and desire to make creative reparation (Klein 1952/1988). Further, in promoting confidence in the container's robustness, the group becomes available for object usage (Winnicott 1971/1974), paving the way, within the group transitional space, for 'freer use of imagination, thought, and feeling, and, in particular, the exercise of play' (Nitsun 1996: 63).

More broadly, the anti-group can be framed within a dialectical perspective: a perspective that sees tension (between opposites) as the basis of transformation:

> A dialectical imagination invites us to embrace contradiction and flux as defining features of reality . . . encouraging us to recognise that the parameters of organisation define the rallying points for disorganisation, that control always generates forces of counter-control, and that every success is the basis of a potential downfall.
>
> Morgan (1986: 265)

Drawing on Ogden (1992a, 1992b), who describes psychopathology as a collapse of this dialectic in one direction, Nitsun (1996) describes anti-group and 'pro-group' as 'two poles of experience that define the development of the group' (p. 204). It is not the presence of the anti-group that is pathological but a collapse of the dialectic in the direction of destructive processes. Similarly, a collapse in the direction of pro-group cohesive forces, leaving destructive forces denied, split off and projected, also threatens development. Thus, from this dialectical perspective, the matter is no longer Bion versus Foulkes but Bion *and* Foulkes as group analysis becomes 'a way of dealing with Eros and Thanatos in an endless ebb and flow' (Cortesao 1991: 271).

Other 'other' approaches

For reasons of both brevity and bias, any overview is prone to omissions. Amongst the most significant is the limited reference to contributions from outside psychoanalysis. For example, historically, a fuller account would include the influence of systems theory (Bertalanffy 1968; Miller 1969; Bateson 1972) and its continued elaboration in the work of Agazarian (Agazarian and Peters 1981; Agazarian and Gantt 2000). Although the 'systematic dialogue' with systems-oriented group therapists that Foulkes hoped for never emerged (Durkin 1983), the influence of systems thinking, being present from the start in Goldstein's work on the neuronal network, though rarely explicit, has been pervasive. Readers interested in pursuing these ideas are directed to Blackwell's (1994) useful introduction as well as more recent discussions (Brown 2003; Gantt and Hopper 2008a, 2008b; Schermer 2012a, 2012b).

Two radicalising challenges to mainstream group analysis also demand brief reference, namely Dalal's post-Foulkesian perspective (1998, 2001, 2002) and Stacey's theory of 'complex responsive processes' (2000, 2001, 2003, 2005).

Radicalising Foulkes

Dalal's distinction between orthodox and radical Foulkes has already been briefly mentioned (see Chapter 4). Allying himself with the latter, Dalal draws more deeply upon the work of Elias (1939/2000, 1989/1991; Elias & Scotson 1965/1994). Thus the 'individual' mind is construed not only as being formed by the social nexus in which it develops (an Eliasian idea Foulkes readily adopts) but that social nexus is characterised by social power relations (an idea that Elias emphasises but Foulkes does not). It is these power relations that profoundly influence how we think about, experience and relate to ourselves and each other.

The social unconscious, in which power relations are both enshrined and denied, feeds our assumptions about difference, allowing groups to use power to reinforce their dominance over other groups. A central, radical, post-Foulkesian task then is to pursue awareness of the dynamics of the social unconscious: 'progressively to stand outside the context we are inside in order to scan it, to enter another context, ad infinitum' (Brown 2003: 159). In response, however, Hopper (2002), though appreciating the need to 'be sensitive to the constraints of the external world', suggests that:

> We must not adopt an overly socialised model of man without instincts, drives, sensations and physiology, not to mention passion, who is merely a figment of the imagination of powerful others. I would not like to be a patient of a group analyst who regarded people in this way.
>
> Hopper (2002: 334)

Complexity theory

Stacey draws on complexity sciences (Nicolis and Prigogine 1989) as a 'source domain' for analogies and, translating these into human terms using the work of social psychologists Mead (1934) and Elias (1989), and 'language psychologists' Bhaktin (1986) and Vygotsky (1962), elaborates the Foulkesian idea that individual minds and social relationships arise together. Again, in accord with radical Foulkes, there is no room for 'internal' (the inner world of the individual) or the 'external' (the outer world of society) – not separately. However, whilst Foulkes appears content to modify internal world psychoanalytic concepts such as the unconscious, transference and countertransference to meet a more socially contextualised perspective, Stacey recasts them as forms of 'complex responsive processes'. Projective identification, containment and even the matrix share the same fate.

Behr and Hearst (2005), though broadly appreciative of this 're-working' – foregrounding as it does the importance of communication, of evolving patterns of interaction, of the illusory nature of separating inner from outer – question its absolutism and suggest its unrelenting translation of psychoanalytic theory into the more elaborate language of complex responsive processes potentially diminishes, rather than revitalises, the processes it describes.

Conclusion

The journey this brief introduction has taken, from group analysis's conceptual birth in Goldstein's neurological post-WWI studies, to its recent radical twenty-first-century elaboration in the wake of complexity sciences, has been a long, winding, though necessarily adumbrated one. Characterised by a spirit of eclecticism, its efforts to 'accommodate' theoretical diversity can, at times, threaten cohesion.[4] Yet, despite this diversity, a fundamental coherence remains; one rooted in the principle of interconnectedness, in a profound, shared understanding that group and individual are inextricably entwined.

Notes

1. This slightly mischievous subtitle is not intended to suggest there are only two therapeutic approaches to groups or indeed only two psychoanalytically informed approaches. Nevertheless, in the UK at least, two psychoanalytically based group approaches do predominate: group analysis and, based on the work of Bion, the Tavistock model. In this context then, the term 'other' intimates a complex historical rivalry between the 'schools'; one which, though having its source in real and significant differences, has also, I believe, been complicated by the dynamic processes of splitting and projection.
2. Hopper (2009) notes a similarity between baO and massification. One might also link 'aggregation' and baM. Indeed, Cano (1998) suggests baO and baM function 'alternately and indifferently'. She thus re-formulates baO and baM as one basic assumption: basic assumption Grouping (baG). A group in the throes of this baG fantasises total union or total self-sufficiency instead of wrestling with the painful, risky business of trying to achieve realistic interdependence.
3. Smith and Berg (1988) note that it is well nigh impossible to have a group devoid of conflict since contradictory processes of progression and regression, individuality and belonging, attachment and alienation occur in tension in most groups. In therapy groups, where members are more likely to experience relational difficulties, such conflict may be even more acute. Nitsun (1996) also identifies ten group analytic group characteristics that can aggravate tensions and stimulate, in response, the anti-group (pp. 48–54).
4. That two prominent group analysts, Vella (1999) and Stacey (2000, 2001), bridging the millennium, envisage very diverse approaches to group analysis – the latter challenging its psychoanalytic foundations, the former arguing a return to Freud – nicely captures the strain on group analytic cohesion that diversity brings.

Part 3

Group music therapy

Developmental perspectives

Chapter 8

Early years
Experiences with others

Alison Davies

I focus on the beginnings of life in this chapter because an understanding of early development in the dyadic relationship between mother/carer and baby helps us to see how relationships grow and develop throughout life in the social world that we all belong to. As therapists, especially music therapists, this is very relevant because much of the work focuses on pre-verbal or non-verbal experience.

In the early months of social development mother and baby share a language of sound and facial gesture. During the first three months of life the baby's responses are mostly in the form of movement, but from then on the baby's communicative repertoire begins to encompass vocalisations and facial expressions. This facial engagement becomes a sort of playful socialisation and the dyad of baby and mother becomes a rich partnership.

In relation to all that the mother/carer does to help the child learn at this early stage, Stern (2010) writes:

> The list includes what you do with your eyes when with another, how long to hold a mutual gaze, what turn-off head movements work, and with whom, how close you should let the other come to you and at what speeds (or you to them, and what distance for whom), what you do with your face (and with whom), how to kiss, how to read body positions, how to solicit another for food, for physical contact, or to play, what the rules of 'peek-a-boo' or 'I'm gonna get-cha' are, how to enter into turn taking when vocalizing with another, how to greet or not greet your mother for a reunion when she returns after a separation, and, how to joke around, negotiate, escalate, back off, and express affection, make friends, and so on.
>
> Stern (2010: 110–11)

These are all important aspects of learning that involve forms of vitality, to be explored in the course of this chapter.

The development of a language which is shared interpersonally between mother and baby is the basis of an ability to relate. For example, Stern (2010: 111) speaks about the understanding of a relationship at this stage that allows each partner to know that the other is fully 'there'. The mother and baby couple recognise the uniqueness of each other's movements and learn, for instance, the emotional feel of each other, such as when and how they get angry or when they are fully attentive or not. Christopher Bollas (2000), describes the mother who

> bathes the infant in seductive sonic imagery, ooing, cooing and aaahing, luring the infant's being from autistic enclave into desire for this voice. As the mother words her infant's gestures, with the onomatopoetics of 'oohing' and 'aaahing', she extends his or her body through this sonic imagery, which is maternal parole.
>
> Bollas (2000: 43)

The music of the mother's vocal interactions leads and releases the infant into the world of communication and ultimately into the world of words.

Of importance at this time is the intensity of stimulation, whether it is visual, auditory, tactile or, what Stern calls, an 'intensity of expectation' (2010: 107). The stronger the stimulus, the more the infant has to regulate, turn away from or reject the source of stimulus. The baby might, in this instance, appear to engage but in real terms switch off or turn away as if to reduce the impact. This can sometimes be seen in a baby crying from overload. Alternatively if the stimulus is too weak and does not arouse the baby enough, the baby may become uninterested, inattentive or fall asleep. Parents have to be tuned in to the nuances of these responses in order to adjust to the baby. Of interest to the music therapist is the fact that these aspects of early attentiveness and the developing of a store of feeling responses, often in musical sounds, could set the patterns of relatedness for the future. All these approaches use the energy of vitality affects.

Vitality affects

Vitality affects are part of human experience: the experience of aliveness. We all have a sense of ourselves and each other through the energy of vitality whether it is through emotions or states of mind. Vitality affects are present in dynamic forms in all the time-based expressive arts where the vitality that is expressed by one person resonates with another. The group analyst Louis Zinkin (1991) speaks of vitality affects not being able to be grouped in the field of readily available emotions such as anger, sadness, joy, fear, or disgust but rather being understood as more kinetic qualities such as exploding, fading away, accelerating, and so on.

> Vitality affects seem to me like the musical signs that are not the notes to be played but indicate how they are to be played. The musician learns the shape of a crescendo, diminuendo, sforzando, calendo, subito piano, accelerando, con fuoco, allegro ma non troppo and even 'con amore'.
>
> Zinkin (1991: 52)

Characteristics of vitality affects of the kind identified by Zinkin are present in all music, and thus in the improvisations that take place in music therapy.

Stern (2010) identifies five dynamic events that constitute the experience of vitality. These are 'movement, time, force, space and intention/directionality' (2010: 4). 'Movement' and 'force' constitute energy which is dynamically or energetically expressed in time, force, space and direction or intention. Stern points out that movement does not happen in isolation when experienced in the mind.

> It [movement] carries along with it other events. A movement unfolds in a certain stretch of time, even if that is very short. There is a temporal contour or time profile of the movement as it begins, flows through and ends. Therefore a sense of time, its shape and duration is created in the mind along with the movement.
>
> Stern (2010: 4)

This could equally be a description of the passage of time in music.

Stern describes vitality forms as the very basis of the experience of feeling in connection with other people. He argues that 'dynamic forms of vitality are the most fundamental of all felt experiences when dealing with other humans in motion' (2010: 8).

Exploring the nature of forms of vitality returns us to the earliest of experiences and Stern (2010: 10) draws attention to the 'in utero' experience of the unborn child. He describes foetal behaviour as important in the development of 'the arousal system' as preparation for the unfolding of forms of vitality.

As early as five to six weeks after conception, in the movement and flexing of the foetus, arousal activities can be observed. This may be due to the sensitivity of the foetus to stimuli, or it could be the earliest glimmer of vitality forms. Stern (2010) talks about generalised movements of the foetus at about three months and from then on as partial movements or gestures such as touching body parts, turning the head, or opening the mouth. Distinguishing these gestures from reflexes, Stern describes these specific movements as clearly not stereotypical but as 'soft assembled' and 'the result of spontaneous activity in the arousal centres that trigger different body parts, which are assembled in slightly different patterns depending on the physical conditions at that moment' (2010: 102).

Of particular interest to the music therapist is how the foetus reacts to the voice of the mother. Experiments transmitting both the mother's voice and then another woman's voice at the same pitch, through the umbilical chord of the baby in utero, have shown that at birth the baby can recognise the particular and unique voice of the mother.

Referring to a research project, Stern (2010: 104) writes:

> At about 6–7 months of gestation, when the foetus begins to perceive external sounds, either one of two melodies is played (experiment 1), or alternatively

the mother's voice or another woman's voice saying exactly the same words (experiment 2) is played to the foetus (i.e to the belly of the mother). This is done every day for months. Then, right after birth, the neonate, only hours old, shows that he can recognise the melody or voice presented to him while still a foetus.

> DeCasper and Fifer (1980); DeCasper and Spence (1986), cited in Stern (2010)

Stern calls these reactions of the foetus 'felt aliveness' rather than vitality forms at this early stage of development.

A clinical vignette

An elderly man with dementia whose attention is very hard to engage, even with music, turns away from the source of sound, closing his eyes and screwing his face up in rejection. He then looks away, out of the window and appears to be somewhere else. As this dementia patient displays aspects of returning to early infantile responses, the music therapist working with him might well think in terms of early affect attunement, adjusting the sound, pitch or dynamics of the music being offered to him or the stress or patterns of rhythms being played. The therapist calls on her ability to respond intuitively to the vitality forms necessary to engage with the patient.

Stern (2010) writes of 'prosody', which he describes as the flow of vitality forms. He is referring to such dynamics as intonation, emphasis and stress patterns of rhythms etc. These are all musical elements that the mother experiments with in order to expand the interest and the engagement of the baby. What is provided can be described as variations on a theme and helps to keep the baby at a level of arousal. If the same stimulus is repeated too many times without variation it might cause the baby to break off interest. The mother needs to adjust the vitality or energy and vary the stimulus to keep the social interaction alive. This happens often in games such as tickling the baby, where the voice can vary from a growing crescendo to an alert anticipation of unexpected gesture. Timing is important, as is an awareness of the baby's response to over- or under-stimulation. All these interactions demonstrating an energy flow between mother and baby are opening up the developing nervous system to an awareness of social interaction and preparing the infant to live and respond to others in a social world.

These forms of vitality are crucial for the baby to experience or be acquainted with as they form the essential pre-speech vocabulary necessary before spoken language begins to develop. Babies thus learn the flow of dynamic and social interaction with another person and the interpersonal social behaviours that this requires, before the complication of words. Music therapists work a great deal at this pre-verbal stage of infancy, either in helping to stimulate language for children where it is delayed or, at the other end of the spectrum, helping patients to return to a non-verbal, feeling state. An example of the latter might be with an over-articulate adult, where words mask or get in the way of the underlying affect or trauma which might have its origin in a pre-verbal experience or feeling state perhaps way back in infancy.

Affect attunement

Another way of looking at vitality forms is through affect attunement or the matching of forms of vitality. This is a form of harmonising, where the mother tries to blend her responses and behaviour to the quality of vitality that is expressed by the baby. It is interesting to note here that, for the music therapist, like the mother, affect attunement is an important dynamic to understand and to be able to incorporate in the therapeutic alliance. It is also very much a part of what is flowing between people in musical improvisation. The very word attunement has a musical resonance.

Affect attunement is the basis of empathy, and so of great interest to the therapist. Empathy, expressed very simply, is the ability to put oneself in another's shoes. To empathise is to seek to connect with another's emotions and to respond with an appropriate feeling. Simon Baron-Cohen (2003) describes empathy as more of a feminine attribute and in this context we can closely link it with mothering or care giving. He writes:

> Empathizing leads you to constantly search people's tone of voice and to scan people's faces, especially their eyes, to pick up how they might be feeling or what they might be thinking. You use the 'language of the eyes' and intonation as windows to their mind. And empathizing drives you to do this because you start from the position that your view of the world may not be the only one, or the true one, and that their views and feelings matter.
> Baron-Cohen (2003: 22)

Kenneth Wright (2009) emphasises the idea of being 'touched' in relation to empathy. In the early days and months of life, actual touch is the central point of communication between mother and baby. The baby is held, stroked, cuddled, changed, and wiped, all involving touching the skin. But the mother who smiles and laughs, gestures, and plays with him also adapts to the baby. This is another way of being in touch, which creates a mutual emotional response between mother and baby. For Wright, this is the 'experiential reference point for all later experiences of being in touch' (2009: 20).

A mother who can deeply connect emotionally in response to the baby opens the baby up to a mutual shared resonance. If all goes well, the baby learns by first receiving an empathic understanding from the mother, who shows she understands at a deep emotional level. The baby's experience is first matched emotionally by a resonance in the mother. He then knows, at an emotional level, that what he is feeling is understood, felt and received by her; there is a mutual connectedness. The importance of affect attunement and empathy is that the mother then translates her perceived feeling about the baby into her own words or her own language of response. Stern (2010) puts it like this:

> In affect attunement, the mother matches the dynamic features of how the baby acted. This assures the baby that she grasps what he did. However, she does not match the content or modality of the infant's action. Instead she makes her own choice of modality and content. This assures the baby that she understood, within herself, what it felt like to do what he did. It is not an imitation, because she put it 'in her own words' – it carries her signature. It is something she felt, too. She wants a matching of inner states.
>
> Stern (2010: 114)

Most parents do this naturally and spontaneously. It is an important development towards the socialising of the child both within the family and in the outside world. The baby learns how to regulate his or her response with another person and in this is learning about social and cultural boundaries. The developing infant's empathic sensitivity and acquisition of social awareness is an important milestone in a group context, whether it be the family, school, or in due course the many other group arenas that are encountered in life.

What is important about both vitality forms and affect attunement is the connectivity and sense of aliveness to the other person that is created. The communication from the mother is a constant ongoing search to connect inter-subjectively with the baby and to try and understand his 'being in the world'. When the mother 'matches' the baby by gestures such as imitation, the baby can be secure in the knowledge that she is on his wavelength and connected to his emotional state.

Research has shown that after about three months, when up to this time the mother–baby response has been an exact match within a short delay of time, the infant responds to and is more attracted to what is a near but not a 'perfect' match (Gergely and Watson 1999; Gergely et al. 1995). The infant then begins to learn that this not only has resonance for him but it is also expanding his experience by offering something different. With this the child understands the gradual beginnings of separateness, otherness and a 'me-not-me' in relationships. Referring to other research (Markova and Legerstee 2006) Stern suggests that the response of the mother that is not only dependent upon exact imitation is the most pleasing to the infant, resulting in 'more gazing time at the mother, more smiles, more positive vocalizations and fewer negative vocalizations compared with the condition of contingency or the imitation condition' (Stern 2010: 116).

A music therapist attends to these dynamics when working with patients who may have developmental delay, or experience confusion, or (as in people with autistic difficulties, for instance), be ambivalent in their relating to others. Vitality affects are also a big consideration in other clinical areas such as work with people with dementia, with its potential return to early childhood states, or with patients where over-intellectual functioning obscures access to emotional states. All early responses, vocalisations and interactive speech patterns are, at their source, musical responses and can be mirrored, echoed, and responded to through music.

Wright (2009) emphasises that it is not just that the mother physically mirrors a response to the child, but that in response to the more continuous vitality affects that Stern describes, the mother can create an atmosphere that embraces a more ongoing connection to the being of the baby. The mother is adjusting, harmonising and identifying with the energies and stresses such as excitement, enjoyment, frustration and suspense of the baby and providing an atmosphere and emotional response that tells the baby that she has understood.

> The baby reveals the contour of its 'feeling' through shifts of posture and tension, vocalisations and changes in patterns of breathing ... the mother renders this in external form, *capturing* it in her mini performance.
>
> Wright (2009: 23)

Christopher Bollas (2000) remarks that it is only later that these innumerable single impressions are linked to words, as they 'move from the deepest recesses of the unconscious into pre-conscious and eventually into consciousness' (2000: 43). The mother's speech links to the bodily sense of the child and seems to be the locus of eroticism long before words in their own right are used to express desire. Bollas puts it this way: 'In "voicing over" the infant's body, the mother touches her infant through acoustic fingers, recursive to all conversions from word to body, and likewise accomplishing its reversal, as the body is now put into words' (2000: 43).

As the baby matures and has less physical need for touch, and the gradual separation occurs both physically and mentally between the mother and baby due to the baby's growing independence and mobility, the need to find ways to 'stay in touch' becomes more important. Wright (2009) says: 'Long before words become meaningful, non-verbal communication supplements physical closeness (actual touch) as a line of connection' (2009: 20).

In describing the essence of how the mother attunes to the baby, Wright could be talking about how a music therapist responds and connects musically to that part of the patient that may feel lost and disconnected from others. Echoing the mother's ability to identify with what Wright calls the 'shape' of the baby's experience, the music therapist can glimpse the being-in-the-world of the patient as she responds to the pattern of rhythms, tensions and speed in the music. Just as the baby is nurtured and enhanced within this space as she is responded to and attuned to by mother, so the patient has the potential of being met in the same way by the music therapist. The way the mother internalises the shape of vitality affects, reflects and echoes them back to the baby, often transforming the baby's mode of expression into a different modality, seems to echo much that a music therapist is endeavouring to do in the clinical setting in musical terms.

Wright (2009) puts it like this: 'Often such enactments transform the baby's expressive behaviour into a different sensory modality; they also modulate and vary it, much as a musical theme on one instrument may be taken up and repeated, with subtle differences, by another' (2009: 146).

Transitional objects

This is another milestone in the social development of the child that later, as adults, allows us to make sense of our relationships to each other and the world. The terms 'transitional object' or 'transitional phenomena' were coined by D. W. Winnicott (1951). He studied the relationship between the early 'fist in mouth' of the baby or sucking of the thumb in stimulation, and satisfaction of the oral erotogenic zone, which he refers to as a 'quiet union', and the attachment of the older infant to a special object such as a cloth or a soft toy. Both of these Winnicott calls 'transitional phenomena'; their function is to be a replacement in the form of an 'illusion' for the breast or the mother, a place of comfort or a bridge between inner and outer reality. This comes at a time when the child is beginning to separate from his mother, when he begins to move from a state of complete dependence towards gradual independence. The transitional object is a sort of fantasy object that bridges the gap when mother is absent. It is often described as the first 'non-me' object that the child possesses. As well as an actual object such as a blanket, a transitional object or phenomenon can be a tune or a word that soothes and feels like an aspect of the absent mother.

> An infant's babbling or the way an older child goes over a repertoire of songs and tunes whilst preparing for sleep come within the intermediate area of transitional phenomena, along with the use made of objects that are not part of the infant's body yet are not fully recognised as belonging to external reality.
> Winnicott (1951: 230)

Winnicott goes on to say the experiencing of this intermediate area is contributed to by both inner reality and external life. He describes it as a place that is not challenged, and 'no claim is made on its behalf except that it shall exist as a resting-place for the individual engaged in the perpetual human task of keeping inner and outer separate yet inter-related' (1951: 230).

The acquisition of a transitional object allows the experience of the mother to come alive when the mother is not there. Wright (2009) identifies this as the key to emotional survival and the ability to later contain and hold feelings within oneself.

> first, it is only possible to feel '*in touch*' with feelings that have been contained within a form or an object; and second, feelings can only be *contained* in so far as the means to grasp them symbolically or pre-symbolically (transitionally), are available. *Transitional* containment is the key to emotional survival: *symbolic* containment is the key to holding feelings in mind and getting to know what they are like.
> Wright (2009: 21)

Clinical implications in the music therapy space

The focus on transitional phenomena is important when thinking of the potential of the therapy space and also of the kind of transitional space that might be offered in the group. In the clinical setting the search for a deeper understanding and wish to know the quality of a patient's experience is an essential task of a music therapist and, in her musical response to the patient, reminds us of the early search of the mother to attune to the baby. This is especially true in relation to those patients who have had less than adequate mothering.

Conclusion

If the baby can feel resonated with and the essence of their experience met and understood in a multitude of enriching and varied ways, this provides an essential precursor to spoken language. It is also a rich area for music therapists working, for instance, with children with developmental delay. For others it may be important to be met musically when touching on or revisiting a traumatised area where there may not be words. The music therapist, depending on the capacity for spoken language, or perhaps the need to get to the feeling beyond the words, has often to stay within the non-verbal arena. Thus a patient with little or no spoken language, or where words are inadequate in describing their suffering, can feel met, understood and connected with through music.

I end by looking at how Wright (2009) sees the relevance of these early stages in life in relation to artistic creativity.

> It is a possibility that the richness of the artist's imagination and his skill in finding forms for inner feeling states is a later development of the mother's intuitive skills – or perhaps a compensation for her relative lack of them. In mastering the techniques of his art, the artist has taken over the mother's form-making capacity, and brought it to fruition in his work. Not only does he now make the spontaneous and vital gestures that express his individuality; he also finds in his chosen medium the answering forms that bring them to reality in the objective world.
>
> Wright (1998: 147–8) cited in Wright (2009)

One very important function of music therapy is to help release creativity through connecting and sharing in music; this can be encouraged in a group through the improvising of music together. In this chapter the focus has been on early stages of life and the social implications for the developing child. The dyadic relationship through auditory and musical dialogue sets the scene for all subsequent relationships, including those in groups.

Chapter 9

Music, attachment and the group
Mainly theory

Eleanor Richards

> This play ... is an affirmation of life – not an attempt to bring order out of chaos nor to suggest improvements in creation, but simply a way of waking up to the very life we're living, which is so excellent once one gets one's mind and one's desires out of its way and lets it act of its own accord.
>
> Attributed to John Cage

This chapter sets out to look at some of the main principles of attachment theory, to relate them to some aspects of group analysis, and to consider whether thinking in these terms is helpful when considering group therapy in which we work with music.

Music is innately social. It has its origins in collective social activity; long before the arrival of performance or formal study of method and technique, it was quite ordinarily turned to as a natural means by which to express something of the experience of being together, or simply a routine part of everyday goings-on. In some places in the world, this remains the case. Pavlicevic (1997) describes vividly her experience of walking through a street in a South African city where a group of drummers were playing; local people generally ignored the musicians, or occasionally broke off from their immediate business to join in, whereas non-Africans, by contrast, needed to stop and listen, as if to a performance.

Music seems always to have been associated with its capacity to represent and give voice to our experience of some of the most central elements of our lives, such as religious practice, family and public celebrations, the marking of significant life events or the expression of mourning. There are two important reasons for that, perhaps. Firstly, music can give a voice to feelings and levels of emotional experience not always to be found in words; secondly, music can bring a structural frame through some of its central parameters (rhythm, harmonic idiom, patterns of repetition), which may provide containment for collective experience that may feel potentially overwhelming.

That being so, it is perhaps not surprising that in due course music therapists turned to the thought of collective music making as a means by which to give some voice to the experiences of groups of people together and to investigate the possibilities of group music as a therapeutic medium. Some of the early proponents of music therapy in Britain, such as Mary Priestley, were themselves in analysis of the traditional verbal kind; it seems probable that as they began to consider the nature and meaning of music for themselves, they might have reflected upon its connection with wordless (or unwordable) experience and so begun to consider improvised, 'free associating' music as a potentially powerful means of therapeutic process and exchange.

The fact that music has always been made in groups is to do with more than simply the need for greater volume levels, or the possibility of more elaborate textures; most musicians will describe the emotional and relational satisfaction inherent in making music with others, and in particular the pleasure to be found in unspoken, attuned collaboration. There is pleasure for audiences, too, in sensing the profound and intuitive communications taking place between musicians in all sorts of idioms from a string quartet to free jazz to a cathedral choir. The language of music readily uses words that imply collective experience: one definition of the word 'ensemble' is of 'a group of items viewed as a whole rather than individually' and the word 'concert' itself comes from the Italian 'concertare' – to harmonise. Perhaps the life of a well-functioning, collaborative music-making group offers a model of interaction and shared inventiveness that resonates with us all, and implies the capacity for both confidence in the value of one's own contributions and openness to the communications and resonances of others that are among what Bowlby identified as the characteristics of secure attachment.

Attachment theory has been increasingly discussed in psychoanalytic circles in recent years. It is now readily taking its place as having a clear theoretical basis in relation to other aspects of psychoanalytic thinking, in particular such areas as object relations theory and, importantly for our purposes here, group analysis. Perhaps what distinguishes attachment theory from other aspects of psychoanalytic theory more than anything else is its emphasis upon the place of the individual in an emotional and social context. None of us exists in solitude; none of us can therefore be considered alone. Rather, our sense of who we are and the meaning of that, and of how we are able to perceive ourselves, emerges from that sense of ourselves which we have gained from our experience of being with others.

Attachment theory rests in the conviction that for each of us our sense of autonomy and emotional wellbeing depends upon the security of a place in a network which is characterised, amongst other things, by mutual concern. Marrone puts it like this:

> optimal functioning of individuals and societies is contingent upon the hard-won developmental capacities for sensitive responsiveness, reflective thinking, reciprocal support, deep-seated trust and stability in relationships
> Marrone (1998: 12)

The term 'attachment theory' was coined by John Bowlby; he developed his ideas through a combination of perceptive self-reflection, clinical observation and practice, writing, and research. His interest in attachment from a therapeutic point of view had one of its beginnings in his period of work during the late 1920s in a home for what were then called 'maladjusted' children. There he encountered some children who had committed serious acts of violence and cruelty. He was struck by their charm and intelligence, but also by their extreme difficulty in making lasting friendships; their anxiety about their own survival was so great that they would abandon, betray or attack their apparent friends at the first sign of conflict. As Bowlby began to recognise that many of these children had family backgrounds characterised by violence, abandonment, criminality and poor sexual boundaries, he grew stronger in his conviction that personality development is directly informed and shaped by real-life events in early life.

> Bowlby . . . saw relationships as central from the start of life and strongly disagreed with the prevailing psychoanalytic view at the time of the infant as an 'autistic', unsocialised, self-absorbed creature, only gradually and with great difficulty learning about and accepting the existence of its fellow creatures.
> Holmes (1996: 205)

Marrone considers the implications of that for our developing capacity for relating:

> The individual lives from the moment he is born until the moment he dies in an interpersonal or intersubjective context. In this context he becomes attached to his parents or parental substitutes and a few other people with whom he develops a close relationship. In the course of the experiences he has with these people (or in relation to them, both in their presence and in their absence), he develops mental representations of the quality of these attachment relationships. These mental representations act as organising factors in the individual's intrapsychic world and influence personality development in an optimal or pathological way.
> Marrone (1998: 17)

Bowlby's interest in attachment is often primarily thought about in terms of the possibilities these ideas offer in clinical work with individual patients. Equally, however, his recognition of the essentially social nature of experience brought him to involvement with the Institute of Group Analysis, to supervision of group analysts and to a growing recognition in his own work of the value of thinking in group analytic terms.

Bowlby took the straightforward view that healthy attachments, both in close partnerships or friendships and in groups or networks, are profoundly necessary for human wellbeing. In early life, attachment needs and behaviours have close connections with the need for physical survival. Bowlby found himself very interested in the ways in which young animals, in particular mammals, may mobilise concern and protection from the adults responsible for their care through various gestures such as clinging, crying, following, and so on. In later life it may be our relationships with our peers or with those in our shared networks that become important; although the fear of physical risk does not carry the same strength, our need for the emotional reassurance brought by the availability of attachment figures continues. Bowlby called these 'affiliative' relationships; he recognised, however, that throughout life such relationships exist within, and are characterised by, an intricate network of representations and understandings.

Perhaps what distinguished Bowlby's thinking most sharply from that of many of his contemporaries in the developing world of British psychoanalysis in the mid-twentieth century was his emphasis upon the significance and impact of early trauma rooted in actual events. This interest in the impact of real-life experience brought him to be, to some great extent, at odds with such thinkers as Melanie Klein who chose to root her understanding of psychopathology far more in the infant's struggle to manage unconscious fantasy. Bowlby therefore found himself most at ease in the so-called Independent Group within the British Psychoanalytical Society, sharing with others such as Balint, Fairbairn and Winnicott the conviction that our emotional difficulties throughout life lie in the first place in difficulties in our interpersonal relations rather than, as Klein might suggest, in the struggle to manage the conflict between our own internal impulses. For Bowlby, therefore, any psychoanalytic endeavour must concern not the study of the individual in isolation, but consideration rather of the individual in her social and interpersonal emotional context.

Bowlby's experience of working with young people who had committed serious and violent acts contributed directly to his conviction that all sorts of psychological problems may derive from a sense of early deprivation. At its most basic that may take the form of unmet physical needs – lack of nourishment or undue physical risk – but just as profoundly it may be to do with a lack of sufficient emotional availability from the caring adults. Psychological health is dependent upon a sense of continuing responsiveness, understanding and support from important others. Without that fundamental security, management of relationships in the later stages of life may prove difficult. At the very least it may lead to situations in which the sufferer experiences anxiety, self-doubt, or depression; in circumstances of even greater difficulty it may be that satisfying relationships and friendships prove impossible to establish or sustain. In discussion with professional colleagues during the 1960s, Bowlby was particularly struck by some of the thinking of R.D. Laing, with its suggestion that certain kinds of difficult family relationship may actually generate pathology. It was during 1980s that he took part in seminars at the IGA, and it became clear to him that attachment theory and group analysis share some fundamental principles. Central to this is the view that 'what is going on within an individual is primarily a matter of what is represented from an interpersonal and social web' (1998: 28).

So what did Bowlby himself say about attachment? Here he is in 1977:

> What for convenience I am terming attachment theory is a way of conceptualising the propensity of human beings to make strong affectional bonds to

particular others and of explaining the many forms of emotional distress and personality disturbance, including anxiety, anger, depression and emotional detachment, to which unwilling separation and loss give rise.

Bowlby (1977: 44)

Bowlby proposed that psychoanalysis should concern itself above all with the study of emotional life and relationships (this seems very familiar to all those working with groups). It places him at some distance, however, from those theories that put such issues as the death instinct or the resolution of fantasy-driven internal conflicts at the centre of human behaviour. That brings us to another of the central differences between the proposals of attachment theory and, by extension, its broader connections in object relations theory, as well as, by contrast, the implication of what is sometimes called drive theory. Drive theory, as represented in some early thinking of Freud, suggests that our dealings with others are driven primarily by our need to satisfy certain fundamental appetites, most particularly our need for food and for erotic or sexual satisfaction, and that our relations with other human beings take place primarily in order that those needs should be met and our individual survival therefore ensured. If these are seen as the primary drives, that reduces our need for the warmth and assurance generated by emotional relationships to some secondary place. Attachment theory, by contrast, suggests that what is most important is our need for emotional security and for a sense of the possibility of flexible, imaginative interaction with others. That brings it into immediate connection with some of Foulkes' most familiar thinking.

Our attachment behaviours emerge from whatever are our internal representations of relationships. Each relationship that we experience in the early part of life has a specific quality; our sense of it is linked to a specific person. Furthermore, our sense of that relationship is lasting; it may continue throughout our life even after the relationship itself has ended. It has emotional qualities; and it carries specific meanings. Bowlby thought in terms of what he called 'developmental pathways' (Marrone 1998: 41); he suggested that at birth the infant may have an infinite number of possible pathways that she might pursue in terms of developing attachment patterns and understandings; the pathways that actually emerge are determined by the nature of the interactions between the child and her environment. For most of us our earliest relational experience is with our parents and other family members; for those who grow up in circumstances of security and emotional stability, the prospect in later life of developing mature and successful adult relationships is strong; for those for whom early experience has been less advantageous, the possibilities of successful adult relating may be less available.

Mary Ainsworth, who worked closely with Bowlby in researching aspects of attachment patterns, developed through her work the proposal that what is most conducive to secure emotional development is to do with what might be called 'sensitive responsiveness'. Most immediately, that has to do with the parent or caregiver's attunement to the baby's signals; the parent must be available to notice, to seek to interpret, and to respond to the infant's gestures. More difficult emotional circumstances for the young child may not be specifically to do with actively neglectful or abusive treatment, but simply related to circumstances in which the caregiver is less able to attune to or read the infant's mental states, or may not be able readily to support the infant in pursuing her emotional goals. All the way through life, we continue to need emotional responsiveness from those with whom we engage in order to enable us to have a sense of self-organisation and self-worth, and to develop some faith in the possibility of cooperative and reciprocal relating. When the caregiver has not been able to be so sensitive, however, the child may learn that her gestures are ineffective, or perhaps even likely to result in negative outcomes, leaving her feeling at odds with herself and uncertain of her value at the moment when she is most in need of recognition and support.

Life in a group is full of opportunities for our current experiences of relating to be manifested in our assumptions and expectations about our dealings with others, and therefore in the nature of those dealings themselves; it also offers the opportunity to consider how those dealings may be acted out in the group's process of being together, and for reflective thought between group members about understandings of what may be taking place.

Bowlby proposed that each of us develops a set of what he termed 'internal working models' to act as both representations and reference points for understanding of our place in the world. These models, formed early in life on the basis of the experience of early interactions, may become established as influential structures of understanding and cognition which both influence and drive each individual's assumptions and expectations about life in relationship with others.

> Each individual builds working models of the world and of himself in it, with the aid of which he perceives events, forecasts the future and constructs his plans. In the working model of the world that anyone builds, a key feature is his notion of who his attachment figures are, where they may be found, and how they may be expected to respond. Similarly, in the working model of the self that anyone builds, a key feature is his notion of how acceptable or unacceptable he himself is in the eyes of his attachment figures.
>
> Bowlby (1973: 203)

Bowlby's proposal (developed by Ainsworth) of the four now-familiar attachment categories – secure, avoidant, preoccupied and disorganised – has become well known and widely used, and the terminology has been adopted by groups of professionals beyond the therapeutic world, such as psychologists, social workers, probation staff and teachers. On one level that is welcome, and it has contributed to the recognition and application of attachment-based and relational ideas in some important areas of the human services. It has brought with it, however, the risk that these are seen as diagnostic categories, when in fact Bowlby is describing something often much more fluid. It suggests a language that can help us to reflect on the quality of particular relationships or interactions, and to think about their roots in terms of conscious and unconscious experience. Fairbairn takes these thoughts further and suggests that not only is our model of ourselves and our relation to the world developed in this way, but the mind itself is structured by 'the subjective experiences of relational meanings' (Hall 2007: 16). Again, this emphasises a key distinction between the thinking of attachment theory and that of clinicians working within a more Kleinian tradition: in the latter the child may be seen as trying desperately to manage destructive impulses derived from within the self by turning them outward through a process of projection and then developing defences against the 'badness' now inherent in the other; attachment theory, by contrast, sees the infant's relations with others, its styles and patterns, as emerging from pre-verbal experience of the quality and nature of specific relationships. It is important to emphasise that what is represented in each case is not simply the parent or other caregiver as a separate person, but rather the relationship itself.

Much psychoanalytic theory has in common its recognition of anxiety and its associated defences as a central issue in understanding and seeking to develop personality. Bowlby shares that view, but chooses to emphasise that he sees anxiety as primarily a response to the threat of loss and corresponding increase of insecurity in attachment relationships. That relates not only to the possibility of actual loss, such as through bereavement or separation, but to continuing fear of threat to psychological survival through isolation or a sense of worthlessness.

The parent–infant pair is, for almost all of this, our earliest experience of relatedness, and many discussions of attachment start at this point. This suggests that the child's earliest sense of security is achieved through some of the qualities that first dyad makes available. Beyond that, however, most of us soon move into some experience of group life – first in the family, then in a neighbourhood, or being in a class at school – so thinking about attachment must take into account not only the characteristics of individual relationships but the complexities of experience within all sorts of groups. So it becomes the case that not only individual relationships may offer security or insecurity, but that the group as a whole has its own attachment associations. The child will experience patterns of interaction (normally in family life first) which become familiar in certain group situations; recurring experiences of familiar scenarios are then internalised in the form of assumptions and beliefs about what can be expected. Within that, each member of a group may bring particular personal perspectives, but the group as a whole may also seek to develop a shared belief (more or less truthful) about what they are like and how they function. To look at this in rather exaggerated terms for a moment, one family may seem outgoing and adventurous, able to talk openly without too much concealment and be supportive of one another. In another there may be a climate of mistrust, secrecy and fear of violence or other mistreatment and a sense that family members cannot readily look to one another for personal support. Such experiences will be brought by members into the therapy group and may inform, both consciously and unconsciously, their expectations of what is possible, what is forbidden, and how the group will go.

Attachment-based thinking in therapy also emphasises the two-directional or multi-directional nature of the working relationship: In group analysis all the group members, including the therapist, are open to change through the group experience; in the same way, attachment-based thinking implies a situation in which the process can move in both directions. This has its model in early relating: As the child grows up she may gain great security not only from learning that she has access to her carer's attentive and would-be empathic responses to her feelings, but also from the realisation that she is able to offer something of the same kind in return, and that it is that mutuality which allows for growth and new experience. Her repertoire grows and changes, and so does her carer's. Security comes not simply from feeling safe in the hands of the stronger 'other', but more maturely from the recognition that partners in a relationship may sustain one another on equal terms, albeit in different ways. Similarly, Harris (1992, cited in Marrone 1998: 67) makes useful distinctions between different kinds of availability. She suggests that what engenders security is not simply the availability of help in a crisis, but rather the knowledge that one inhabits an emotional climate in which consistent concern and interest are present. She also suggests that the young child experiences the 'absence' of the other not simply when she feels ignored, but also at moments where the other responds with misunderstanding or misplaced emphasis. (Stern might call this 'misattunement'.) For instance, those responding may simply point out the sufferer's own responsibility for her discomfort, or minimise the extent of feeling, or adopt a rather distant role offering no more than practical solutions.

Marrone (1998: 71) says of working models that they are 'cognitive maps, representations, schemes or scripts that an individual has about himself . . . and his environment'. These models can vary greatly in complexity but the common characteristic is that they form a representation ('map') of experience. That may be of a single continuing relationship, past or present, of a recurring interpersonal situation, or of some broader sense of the person's self and his place in the world. They function as a means of organising both subjective and objective experience. A working model has two particular areas of application for each of us. Firstly, it gives some sense of whether our attachment figures or the people in the wider group can or cannot be expected to be responsive; secondly, it indicates whether the person sees himself or herself as someone to whom others are likely to respond. The term 'model', incidentally, which may appear somewhat mechanistic, nonetheless brings with it some advantages, particularly perhaps in its implication that it is something that has been constructed and that therefore, like any structure, is open potentially to modification. So there is something of a paradox: these models can be experienced as stable and dependable, but at the same time they are, in the right circumstances, flexible and open to change.

These distinct yet interdependent models are generally held outside conscious experience, yet they function for any of us as the basis for how we may instinctively forecast how accessible and responsive others may (or may not) be when we turn to them.

For those for whom early family experience has been unfulfilling or has actually brought mental or physical suffering, the prospect of becoming part of a new group, such as a therapy group, may be at best uninspiring and at worst frightening. Earlier groups have not been experienced as sources of understanding or hope; why should this be any different? Foulkes points out that there is also a powerful broader social dimension to anxiety about groups. He suggests (writing in the 1950s) that:

> Modern circumstances tend also to conceive, and treat, the individual as expendable. Plans are made discounting literally millions of human lives without hesitation. No wonder the modern individual is afraid of the group – is afraid of losing his very existence, of his identity being submerged and submitted to the group. The individual, while helplessly compressed into a mere particle of social groups and masses, is at the same time left without any true companionship in regard to his inner mental life.
>
> Foulkes (1957: 24)

At the same time Foulkes turns regularly, in language familiar to musicians, to musical metaphors to sustain his central proposal that wholly individual experience is an illusion; any emotional experience, although distinct to the individual, takes place within a network – in the moment or internally represented (or both) – of relationships.

> If we hear an orchestra playing a piece of music, all the individual noises are produced each on one particular instrument; yet what we hear is the orchestra playing music ... Not even in terms of pure sound do we hear a simple summary, a summation of all the individual waves which reach our ears, but these are modified significantly, being part and parcel of a total sound. In truth what we hear is the orchestra. In the same way mental processes going on in a group under observation reach us in the first place as a concerted whole.
>
> Foulkes (1957: 25–6)

Chapter 10

Music, attachment and the group
Mainly practice

Eleanor Richards

> I'll play it first and tell you what it is later.
>
> Attributed to Miles Davis
>
> Sometimes you have to play a long time to be able to play like yourself.
>
> Attributed to Miles Davis

Making music together is one of the ways in which human beings have related to one another and marked and enjoyed some of the experiences distinctive to being in a group. It also, of course, brings the body into action, and calls for physical as well as emotional engagement (if the two can be separated) with whatever transactions are taking place. There are some pictorial representations in mediaeval manuscripts of monks, for instance, singing together; they stand in a circle and, strikingly, some may have a hand lightly on the shoulder of the person next to him, as if confirming through that gesture something of the innate connectedness and collectiveness of what they are doing. Perhaps this is a useful, if slightly remote, parallel with the life of an improvising group in therapy. Here, too, the participants are in a circle, engaged in a mutually interdependent activity in which the musical product is the outcome of an unspoken connectedness. Like those mediaeval singers, those improvising in a therapy group are neither performers nor audience, but simply jointly involved in their collective musical project. This association of a concrete, tangible experience (playing instruments) with an outcome that is a world of sound outside and beyond verbal translation is perhaps a valuable way to bring together elements of the ordinary and the extra-ordinary – or to put it another way: conscious and unconscious experience. Music is often ascribed the capacity to take the listener into some more distant, transcendent area of experience; perhaps the activity of spontaneously creating music can also, however, assert the reality of the link between ordinary events and the discovery of new and deeper meanings.

For any group of people embarking upon improvised music making for the first time it may be a daunting experience. Familiar associations or assumptions can arise: that it requires expertise to play music, that there are definite if unspoken rules about right and wrong, that only music which sounds a certain way is going to be acceptable or even bearable, that one might by one's own contribution 'spoil' something that was otherwise going well or simply that doing something so unfamiliar with and in front of others feels awkward or dangerous. For some people, too, there may be awkward associations with music at other stages of life, perhaps linked to a sense of failure at school or just a fear that this kind of activity is itself 'childish'. The near-universal professionalisation of music performance leaves many people faced with fears of incompetence or unworthiness. All these anxieties, which contribute to the structure of each person's internal working model, are potentially to be worked with and explored as a means towards greater self and group understanding.

If the group can reach a point of beginning tentatively to 'play' (in every sense), then there may be wider possibilities. One of the pleasures of free collaborative play is that of responding to and taking up ideas that come from someone else, whilst also feeling free to propose contributions of one's own, all the while not quite knowing where the play is going. (That is one of the delights of good conversation.) The confidence to engage with others in that way has its roots in sufficiently secure attachment. The secure child will come out with new ideas in the assurance that her caregiver, and later her peers, will meet them with interest and creative imagination. She will also be able to tolerate those moments at which her ideas are not at the forefront, and will be able to allow and feel interest for the activities of others. Through that process she will learn that life with others is not simply social and pleasurable, but actively creative, and that creativity is always in some sense a social act.

Jeremy Holmes puts it like this:

> We discover who we are through our actions and artefacts. Initially, a parental presence is needed to shape the ability of the child to use first his body as an instrument and then to offer the tools of self expression – the spoon to bang . . . Art is . . . always communicative . . . it is always an attempt to get in touch with the self, through an external medium, which in its origins requires the presence of another.
>
> Holmes (2001: 111)

This is a long way from the anxiety of the group member with her fears of humiliation. If one is too worried that one's activity must meet the standards of some stern internalised critic (who may readily be projected into other group members) then where is the possibility of speaking for oneself? It is that uncertainty about whether one's communications will be welcome, together with fears about the actual nature of the response of the other, that characterises more anxious or avoidant patterns of attachment, which may develop in order to regulate the anxiety generated by a loss of security.

Paradoxically, some of the traditional routines and idioms of Western music may have a lot to offer to the improvising therapy group, even if they seem to represent a level of harmoniousness or complexity which the group believes to be impossible. All Western music up to the end of the nineteenth century, and most of what is still familiar today, is characterised by a secure sense of structure. That is generated through, for instance, regular pulse, familiar harmonic progressions, clear patterns of repetition of certain sections, and a process of forward movement, rhythmic and harmonic, which enables the piece to come to a satisfying conclusion. In the course of the nineteenth century (interestingly, at a stage at which cultural life began to develop much more explicit interest in the inner world of the individual) composers began to build a more active developmental energy into their work. In the first movement of a symphony by Beethoven, for instance, the various thematic ideas which have appeared in the opening pages are subjected to intense exploration through such devices as combining them in new ways, putting them in new harmonic contexts, or breaking them down into some of their smaller components which then, in turn, themselves become very powerful. At the end of the movement the ideas usually return in their original form, but we hear them differently because, with them, we have been through the more dramatic and unpredictable experience of the central section. A process like this, though simple to describe, touches upon a fundamental aspect of human experience to do with change. Our attitude to change is ambivalent: it is unavoidable and sometimes welcome, but it also has absolute associations with the unknown and with loss. Creativity involves both growth and destruction: for something new to arise, something familiar must give way.

It is only in last two centuries that, with the rise of the public concert, a custom has developed of providing programme notes for the listener, as if the music cannot be trusted to speak for itself, or the listener needs some non-musical assurance about the meaning of things. But music therapy, like other forms of relational therapeutic practice, seeks to find meaning in gestures themselves of every kind – musical, verbal, bodily – without necessarily any immediate need for 'translation' or clarification.

Brian

Brian arrived as a newcomer in a group whose other members had been working together for over a year. All, including Brian, had in common recurring experiences of brief psychiatric admissions for a range of symptoms. Brian's arrival was greeted with apparent enthusiasm ('it's good to have a new face') but beyond that the group showed little interest in him or his reasons for being there. When that was eventually pointed out by the conductor, Brian observed that he had had the same experience on the ward, where he had sought to ensure that he stayed in the background and had tried to avoid taking part in groups. At the same time he had found the experience painful, not only because he felt alone and isolated, but because it awakened memories of his early family life. He had been an unexpected late child and had struggled at school, where he was bullied. His older siblings had teased him and developed a family 'myth' that he was thick; his parents did little to protect him. In the group, mostly thanks to gentle enquiries from the conductor, the story emerged. It also became clear that Brian's hopes in relation to being in the group went no further than his wish to manage this situation with less distress; he could not at that point feel or voice any desire to be able to act differently. Brian's internal working model, therefore, was one in which he expected others to treat him patronisingly and with disdain, and in which he expected also to see himself as limited and deserving of nothing else. No experience in his childhood had encouraged him either to protest or in any other way to find a voice of his own. In the group, he was anxiously watchful and said little other than to endorse quietly a view expressed by someone else. The group in turn did not question his stance, and spent much of its time recalling events that had taken place before his arrival. When the conductor in due course pointed that out, group members began to recall that in recent months two other new members had arrived, each of whom had left the group after a few weeks after an episode of disagreement. The group claimed to be mystified by all this. One way to look at this might be to suggest that the group as a whole had developed an anxious internal model of itself as destructive; better not to explore those events too closely, and better to ignore Brian than to risk another manifestation of the group's dangerousness.

So what happened in the music? At first the group played carefully, rhythmically and rather quietly and Brian was able easily to fit in without too much exposure. The steadiness of the music, which might have been interpreted as rather unchanging and defensive, in fact offered Brian a feeling of security, which enabled him to find that he was actively enjoying both the overall sounds and the physical experience of using an instrument. He played a small bell, however, which allowed him to be clearly heard although he played it softly, and enriched the musical texture in a way that others enjoyed and responded to. A group member said jokingly 'Are you ringing to ask to be let in?' Brian replied that he had not consciously thought of that, but he realised that he had not expected to feel welcome. Others in the group began to recount their own feelings of anxiety, and through a mixture of talk and short improvisations the group began to move into more dissonant and unpredictable playing. That, in turn, brought more open discussion in which group members could more readily differ and question one another. Those exchanges were not always easy, but attendance at the group improved and both musical and verbal events unfolded more freely. The opportunity to use music allowed the group to explore 'dissonance' in a way contained by the structure and sounds of the music, and to find that their differences might be sources of strong feeling, but also of inventiveness and movement, sometimes articulated by experiment with more edgy, unpredictable rhythms. The group could let go of its anxious sense of its own riskiness and make room for a broader and deeper emotional repertoire. Brian's own playing became bolder and he began to enjoy surprising the group with some of his contributions.

> The task of therapy is not to eliminate suffering but to give a voice to it, to find a form in which it can be expressed. Expression is itself transformation;

this is the message that art brings ... Such a perilous journey needs to be supported by a therapeutic community, a group which can 'hold' both artist/therapist and sufferers alike.

Levine (1997: 15)

For Brian, the initial defensive 'sameness' of the group's music offered some security, perhaps; it is striking, though, that he chose the sound of the bell, which, although it was small and softly played, cut through the surrounding musical sounds and awoke some associations for others in the group. The group's musical and emotional repertoire began to expand, and its broader 'rhythmic' structure became more spacious: long improvisations and routine talk were replaced by shorter and more immediate bursts of music and dialogue.

The stages of the therapeutic and creative processes are the same ... Creation depends upon destruction, a willingness to give up a previous pattern and to experiment with a new form. Letting-go, the experience of emptiness and the emergence of the new characterise the creative as well as the therapeutic processes.

Levine (1997: 23)

Julia

Julia came to the group because she was having recurrent panic attacks, generally to do with her fear of not fulfilling the expectations of her managers at work. She generally perceived herself as competent and self-contained, but as her career developed and she became more senior, she began to struggle with the demands of some of the tasks that were now hers. She could not bring herself to go to anyone for help; that would have meant acknowledging to both herself and someone else that she was not functioning as perfectly as she believed she should. She began to take time off from work because of 'exhaustion'; she spent those times alone at home in a rather frozen state, sleeping or watching television, and speaking to no one.

In her preliminary meeting with the therapist before starting in the group, she described some of these experiences precisely, but with little feeling. When the therapist wondered whether she could have asked for help, she replied that she was not that kind of person, adding 'I'm a closed system'. She said that she had been a happy, solitary child, and that she was used to sorting things out for herself; she did not expect the group to be helpful, but in coming was obediently taking her GP's advice.

The avoidant person is one who finds it difficult to accept, or even imagine, that others may be interested or sympathetic. She may expect her relationships with significant others to be unchanging and uneventful, and she may be perceived by others as emotionally distant. She may be an excellent observer of the behaviour of others, but she does not easily engage in meaningful exchanges. She is unlikely, too, to allow herself awareness of her own emotional experience, preferring an inner apparent 'neutrality', which she may seek to sustain by avoiding any circumstance in which there may be any risk of disturbance. She may often say that she is fine, and while showing polite interest in the feelings of others, be unable to empathise with their experience. She may be outwardly socially skilled, lively, and with a network of colleagues and acquaintances, but that disguises a disconnection from human relationships at a more profound level.

Julia brought something of this picture to the group. She was apparently lively, and could be wittily amusing, and she remembered very accurately group events and the content of group discussions from week to week. It seemed to be a playing out of the role she relied so much upon at work: that of the efficient, likeable administrator. She remained on the edge, however, and even when invited to do so by other group members she could not relate their experience to her own in anything but the most factual terms. On occasions when another member became distressed, Julia shifted her chair back and sat still and tense, looking at her hands. In due course she would offer some practical suggestions.

The music presented Julia with a situation she had not expected. Before coming to the group, she had said to the therapist that she looked forward to the music 'because with music, you know how it's going to go'. In other words, she hoped that the music would bring regularity and consistency and no surprises – a sort of replication of her preferred state of affairs at work and in her emotional world, where she would not encounter anything that her well-developed system of self-regulation could not cope with. Wallin writes of patients whose 'early interactions have been problematic, registering implicitly as a dispiriting bred-in-the-bone understanding of self and others that they cannot easily articulate but also cannot keep from enacting, often to their own disadvantage' (Wallin 2007: 118).

She arrived in the group at a point at which the existing group members had been experimenting increasingly freely with music that was not always 'harmonious' in the conventional sense, and was sometimes loud. She felt alarmed, not only because there was no obvious scheme of things in which she could find a place to be both competent and unnoticed, but because she found the music itself emotionally distressing in a way that she could neither explain nor ignore. At first she tried to avoid the situation by simply sitting out of the improvisations; in due course another group member commented on her observant, distant stance and asked her if she was all right. She surprised herself by saying that the music reminded her of being shouted at by her mother when she made mistakes as a child, and that it was impossible to get both that memory and the music itself out of her head between sessions. That moment of greater emotional freedom also allowed her to say that she liked the sound of the gong that was among the instruments. The group suggested that next time she should play it to start the music off, and she tentatively did so, with a cautious, quiet, steady beat. The group joined her in music that picked up her pulse, allowing her to feel some influence in events, but also slowly raised the volume level before falling back to a gentler ending. Julia found herself moved by the realisation that she was being listened to, and by discovering that she could bear the responsibility of her place in the music; as the sessions proceeded her playing became bolder and freer as she began to trust the prospect that in improvised music there might not be a 'mistake' in an objective sense. That allowed her to respond more spontaneously to musical gestures from others in improvisations, and to allow herself to feel an emotional response when her own playing was heard and answered. (The eighteenth-century composer C.P.E. Bach remarks somewhere that a musician cannot move others unless he himself is moved.) In discussions of the music Julia was sometimes surprised when others were appreciative of her playing, but she also spoke of the relief of finding a place away from words and cognitive order where she could act freely with less of her usual fear of losing human contact as a result. The experience of music making and her deepening feeling of the music, and by extension the group itself, as a source of security, allowed Julia to become more exploratory not only in her playing, but in her verbal exchanges. She began to recount more of her experience and surprised herself by becoming openly upset describing her lonely life at home and her apprehensiveness at work. Bringing that account into words gave it some reality for her (she was less able to put her symptoms down to 'exhaustion') and allowed others to identify with it, ask questions, and simply be sympathetic. In turn, she could use both the music and the talking more openly.

> Play, then, is the operation of imagination, not of fantasy. In a certain sense, we could say that the goal of therapy is to replace fantasy with imagination, to transform psychological space from an isolated lifeless world of private obsessions into a connected, vital field of play. Therapy can then be understood to be a re-vitalization of the imagination, a turning-back to original connection between self and world.
>
> Levine (1997: 33)

Tina

Tina often came to the group in a state of agitation. She worried about all sorts of practical issues – the temperature of the room, whether she could have a glass of water, whether she would miss the bus on the way home – and constantly asked other group members for their advice and reassurance about these things. When she had the opportunity, she would bring stories from other parts of her life which were dramatic or harrowing, or she talked about disasters which were in the news. Often her narratives were fragmented and hard to follow. All of this led others to feel at times that they must attend to her; if the focus in the group was upon someone else or conversation became more general, Tina would become silent and abstracted, or else find a link which could draw the discussion back to her. She was not curious about the wellbeing of anyone else and often did not notice absences until they were pointed out. Not surprisingly, this style led others to become increasingly irritated, so that her anxious need for acknowledgement in fact drove them further away. In the music she sometimes slowed the pace of events by taking a long time to choose an instrument, making the group wait. She found the experience of the music as group event, in which no one might stand out, hard to tolerate; she would play quietly but without engagement, as if waiting for it to be over. It was as though without active endorsement from outside she might not feel assured of her existence or value. At first she was not able to wonder why she needed to mobilise others in this way. Attachment theory suggests that the child gains her capacity for self-regulation from some central elements in early carer–infant interaction: if the carer is preoccupied, or unpredictably absent, physically or psychologically, it is difficult for the child to feel the continuing unfolding of his self-understanding. When things go better '[the carer's] habitual reactions to his emotional expressions focus the infant's attention on his internal experiences, giving them a shape so that they become meaningful and increasingly manageable' (Fonagy 2001: 170). Without such attuned, imaginative responses the child has no one to contain his experience or help him to manage it, and may develop a way of relating that is driven by repeated anxious attempts to be sure of drawing the carer's attention, albeit briefly and superficially. Tina's contributions to the music were not only rather emotionally disengaged and apparently apathetic, but also outside the prevailing rhythmic pulse, emphasising not only her difficulty in being part of an event in which she was not the focus of attention, but also, perhaps, her difficulty in feeling any shared underlying meaning or aesthetic direction in what was happening. After an improvisation in which her detachment from events had been particularly apparent, another group member asked her why, when she so enjoyed dramatic stories and tales of anxiety, her playing was so different. She started to tell a complicated anecdote about her piano teacher at school, but the group brought her back to the question in the moment and she became upset and said 'I don't know what I think'. She added that she found the music awkward because she could see that others were sometimes communicating in it, but she could not imagine how to be part of that. The group suggested that she might try simply fitting in with whatever was going on; one person said 'That'll make you listen'. On one level it could be said that once more Tina had drawn the attention of the group and was getting 'help'; what was suggested, however, was not only in her interests but also in the those of the group as a whole, inviting her to take her place in a gathering of equals. In the next improvisation Tina actively played a steady rhythmic background on a drum; in that and in subsequent music, she began to feel the pleasure of being part of something collaborative, in which she could feel the value of her part in things with less anxiety about being unnoticed or turned away from.

> The aesthetic dimension emphasises the search for a form or container within which feelings can be truthfully symbolized . . . This container may be the analytic relationship itself . . ., art in all its varied forms, or religion.
> Holmes (1996: 189)

Stein (1999) points out that in the conventions of music in the West, understandings of what may be experienced as 'consonant' or 'dissonant' have not remained constant; the mediaeval ear, for instance, might have struggled to tolerate some sounds that are readily accepted now. Harmony itself has become increasingly rich and complex, and since the start of the twentieth century tonality itself has ceased to be the only governing principle, as composers have increasingly sought expressivity and meaning through other forms of harmonic and melodic structure. That, of itself, might be thought of as a large-scale (and continuing) evolutionary or developmental process; our overall personal and social development is reflected in our aesthetic life. New developments are often resisted because of their strangeness; in attachment terms, that might be to say that we may cling to our existing models of experience, however limiting or unsatisfactory, because they offer us some sort of familiarity. It is in the gradually accepted framework of relational security (in the group, for instance) that we may be more able to risk some experimentation or actively search for new and more authentic means of expression and exchange. As some of the clinical material in this chapter implies, it may be that in shared music making some fixed assumptions and patterns of relating can begin to be relaxed more readily at first than through verbal discourse. Freely improvised music can take on a momentum of its own through which, both for the group and for its individual members, the pleasure of finding a developing musical 'repertoire' (or its own 'tonality') which is experienced as adventurous and yet emotionally coherent may translate into the emergence of freer relating and a more secure sense of self and of the possibilities of relational life. Just as the mother and infant develop a subtle, sophisticated mutual language of emotional recognition long before any of it can be described or discussed in cognitive terms, so music itself, and above all the experience of creating it with others, carries an immediacy that is recognisable on a profound level outside cognition. Its emotional content may be contained within familiar structures or idioms, yet, as Schopenhauer suggests, 'the effect of music is so very much more powerful and penetrating than is that of the other arts, for these others speak only of the shadow, but music of the essence' (quoted in Storr 1992: 140). Writing about poetry (but music would do just as well), Holmes says:

> Without an intersubjective perspective people suffering mental pain are stuck – trapped within their narcissism or nihilism (which is only a negative form of narcissism). Psychotherapy and poetry help us escape from this cul-de-sac. Both put us in touch – physiologically, emotionally, cognitively – with creativity and with the living reality of the other.
> Holmes (2002: 139)

To return to Bowlby: his proposal was that our internal working models of ourselves and of our relationships, and our assumptions about 'how things go' are both generated and continually re-enacted outside conscious awareness. Cognitive observation and discussion of them can only take us so far; it is in new relational experience that they may become open to change and greater freedom. Improvised music in the group, offering players the chance to investigate different ways of being in relation to one another through the experience of evolving co-created music, may take them beyond familiar emotional and procedural structures into a place of more open and direct meeting.

Part 4

Group music therapy

Clinical perspectives

Chapter 11

Clinical vignettes

This chapter brings together a collection of brief vignettes drawn from group music therapy practice with a range of client groups. Some reflect free improvisational approaches, with obvious affinities to some aspects of group analysis. Others, however, demonstrate that analytic thinking can be of equal value in informing understanding of group processes in the context of work where group activities are necessarily more structured.

Music therapy with a group of people with dementia

Karen Gold

'I'm going to make a complaint about you,' said B, fixing me with a jokey stare. I swallowed hard, and replied: 'What will you complain about?' She retorted: 'Well you're 30 years too young, for a start.'

In late dementia, primitive feelings – envy, grief, rage, terror – tend to emerge uninhibited. But earlier on, striving to sustain social conventions is both difficult *and* reassuring: a kind of polite scaffolding. So a group analytic approach to therapy – allowing themes to emerge, reflecting overtly on group interaction and unconscious resonance – can seem to threaten the very disintegration people with dementia most fear. It can also bring cohesion, aliveness, intimacy and joy.

The group described here is slow-open. Its four members attend 12 weekly sessions in a pleasant but slightly exposed dayroom whose windows face the hospital car park. They sit in a circle in upright chairs (not armchairs) around a coffee-table with xylophone, glockenspiel and small percussion instruments chosen to mix prompts to memory – tambourine, maracas, cowbell – with prompts to curiosity – kalimba, Indian bells, wooden and metal agogo. On the floor are bass chimes and various hand-drums. There is a guitar and a small piano.

Each week I remind the group that our music and words are confidential, and I end on time. Lengthy hospital appointments, circuitous transport routes, conversational repetitiveness; all are unconscious attempts to imply that older people's time is endless, says Danielle Qinodoz (2010). But of course end*less* is just what older people's time is not.

This account draws on three sessions of an established group of people with moderate (mid-stage) dementia. Names and some details have been changed.

Late April

Grace, 84, a widow, quick as a sparrow, picks up a beater to play a Christmas carol on glockenspiel. She loves church singing, she says, launching into a sultry *Begin the Beguine*. Anita, 77, witty by day but violent at night, joins in. Harry, sardonic, mid-80s, says he has forgotten the words. He taps a beater on his forehead, adding 'What I've got here is terrible.'

Anita asks, 'Is it good to remember things?' Silence. I say, 'What do people think?' Harry and Scandinavian Erik, 81, begin to praise the prettiness of the pergola outside. I say 'It seems difficult for people to stay in here; it seems we're talking about something painful.'

At once the group starts to play. Anita shakes a tambourine, others hit drums and xylophones. Grace's rhythm begins to gallop. I find myself singing Rossini's William Tell overture. At the end I ask Grace what she was thinking of. She says 'Racehorses.' I say 'Start or finish?' She says 'Becher's Brook.' I say 'That sounds a dangerous place.' Harry taps a drum, Anita the xylophone. I say 'You had the last word.' She smiles. There is talk about maybe learning the piano, joining a choir. Grace begins to repeat her xylophone carol, then stops, confused. My stomach tightens. Nobody speaks. The clock ticks. Laboriously she restarts and, hesitating, reaches the end. A little group music breaks out, poignant with relief: glockenspiel glissandi, taps on bass chimes. Erik says, 'I've got this thing, I can't remember the name.' I say 'Do you want me to say it?' He says yes. I say, rather slowly, 'It's Alzheimer's.' Anita says 'Why us?' Grace says 'What will be will be,' adding in song *Que sera, sera*. Erik says he didn't used to be naughty or nasty. I say perhaps they think it's their fault. Anita says yes, fast. Erik says if someone hit him in the playground of course he'd hit them back. I say, 'Perhaps with dementia you can't hit back, you can't give as good as you get.' Erik says he'd like to sing something, from long ago, if people don't mind. There are nods and, in Latin, in tears, he sings the entire *Confiteor*.

Early May

Unprompted, everyone plays energetically; tuned percussion, shakers, tambourines. There is a mutual diminuendo, then crescendo; it feels very connected. As the music finishes, Harry speaks of visiting war graves in France. Someone mentions World War I, the Christmas Day football match before German and British soldiers returned to slaughter. Harry says, angrily, 'It made a mockery of it.' Everyone agrees. I feel sure this is about playing music in the face of dementia, but all I can find to say is 'There's some fear and anger in here.'

Late May (Harry is absent)

A chair is moved, so all three are facing me. What can they do today? they ask. Will I teach them something? 'I thought we'd hear you play lovely music,' adds Erik. 'We all played last week.' I say: 'I think you want something from me that I can't give you.' Grace circles a tambourine around her head, stopping herself, saying 'I've had a good life.' There is talk of memory and Alzheimer's. Then she begins a bongo rhythm, which turns into *The Blue Danube*. We all sing it animatedly to 'la'. There is talk of dancing. Erik stands up, takes a step towards Anita, turns away and demonstrates waltzing alone. He sits down to applause.

I say, 'I thought you were about to ask Anita to dance.' She looks coy. Erik hesitates, says 'I could . . .' holds out his arm to her. They dance. Grace and I sing, Grace watching them intently. Anita sits down, blushing like a girl. There is a glow in the room. Turning to me Grace says, 'Perhaps Erik could dance with *you.*' I blush. Laughter. I say, 'This is about sex, isn't it?' Grace exclaims 'Ooooh,' brightly. Erik says 'This won't go outside here?' I say no. He jiggles in his chair, saying he's past it, but it was exciting. I say the group feels very alive. Then I notice that we have over-run. The group plays, and talks, finally leaving after I have asked them to stop five times.

Boundaries, a focus on unconscious dynamics, and some reticence in answering personal questions all promote the establishment of group members' transference to the group and therapist. Transferences often take the form of anticipating criticism – a projection of individuals' own hatred of their growing incapacity – expressed as musical inhibition, and in particular a pushing of the therapist into the role of teacher and/or judge. Reminiscences of not being allowed to touch, learn or play the piano are frequent, and I choose to play agogo or Indian bells if I feel that going to the piano may reinforce the group's splitting of ability/disability between us. Meanwhile my countertransference often reflects the group's dementia experience: fragmentation, panic, fear of rejection and shame. I find myself thinking: Do I/they have anything worth playing? If I voice (musically or verbally) something too painful, will they all go and never return? As a group, they never have. And yet ultimately, of course, they – and we – will.

Playing together, being together: infants and their carers in music therapy

Alison Levinge

Winnicott is reported to have said in a seminar, much to the surprise of his audience, 'There is no such thing as a baby.' Referring to this comment in a later talk Winnicott explained that what he had meant was that 'whenever one finds an infant one finds maternal care, and without maternal care there would be no infant' (1960: 39).

It is now well established in psychological and neurological thinking that how we develop in the early years of our lives is strongly dependent upon the ways in which we are responded to by our mother and those supporting the process. Successful development is dependent upon the kind of exchanges we have with our environment along with how we respond to the impact it has upon us. Growing up, or in psychological terms developing a sense of self, is dependent upon the ways we are helped to manage our experiences of life and is reliant upon whether we are successfully helped to regulate and manage the feelings we have about what comes our way.

When infants are securely attached to their mothers they can grow up into children who are confident and successful in their interpersonal relationships. The building blocks for this process are formed by the capacity of a mother to attune and adapt to her baby's needs. If for some reason a mother feels depressed or in low mood, this can interfere with her ability to care for her baby. Providing group music therapy for mothers with their children mirrors aspects of a family unit. A mother may find support from other mothers, children may relate to other children, and the therapist can come to represent a grandmother/father figure providing indirect support. Offering a music therapy group can enable mothers and their children to interact, communicate and relate to each other through a medium which is able to reflect and support elements of a mother–infant relationship.

A vignette

Jane had been struggling for some time. Since Thomas's birth, she had become isolated at home and was finding it difficult leaving her house and mixing with others. Nine-month-old Thomas was clearly healthy, but appeared rather subdued and his mother reported that he did not seem to want to be with her. Her health visitor could see that it was hard for Jane to engage comfortably with her baby and this was confirmed when Jane explained that she often felt at a loss. The health visitor suggested that she might attend a music therapy group, explaining that this could be a place where she could feel supported and where Thomas might be able to engage with other children. The purpose of the music therapy group was to provide an environment in which mothers suffering with low mood or postnatal depression and their babies could discover more satisfying ways of being together. The group of five dyads was prepared for a new member and Thomas and his mother were introduced by their health visitor, who was the co-facilitator of the group.

The group

As we begin the hallo song, Jane appears awkward and, looking around the room, finds it difficult to engage with her son. It is also clear that it is difficult for Thomas to sustain eye contact with his mother and when Jane tries to catch his gaze, he moves his head from side to side. As the music continues, Jane is observed gently swaying in time to the song. Feeling this movement, Thomas shifts his gaze from the nearby baby to the face of his mother. She smiles in response and visibly begins to relax. In turn, Thomas fixes his gaze upon his mother's face, drinking her in. There are several more songs which involve mothers interacting in different ways with their babies, and between each one there is space for each mother to reflect on how she is feeling. As the group continues, there comes a moment when it feels the right time to introduce free play. As music therapist, I support the musical expressions by improvising on the piano, creating a musical container in which mothers and their babies can explore and play in different ways and with whoever feels comfortable. During this time, Thomas is seen crawling away from his mother over to another baby who is playing with a shaker. Meanwhile, Carol, who is sitting next to Jane, looks over toward her, and feeling confident and supported by the improvised music, blows the horn which she has been playing to her daughter and laughs. As if Jane cannot help herself, she picks up another horn and responds, playing tentatively, alternately blowing with Carol's note. The sound is loud enough to attract the attention of the other four mothers and their children and different blowing instruments are found and a 'blowing piece' of music created. The different noises provoke laughter, and some of the babies look surprised and bemused. Following this lively and energetic musical moment there is pause for thought and reflection. Having been able to let go of some of their inhibitions, some of the more confident mothers chatter in animated tones about their experiences of playing in such a free way. Others are quieter, and more withdrawn. The mothers who feel more confident are able to share something of their ambivalent feelings about playing freely, as well as some of the observations they have made of their babies. Following this lively piece of music, I introduce a quieter, more rhythmically based song. All the mothers now hold their children on their laps and gently move back and forth in time to the song. The atmosphere becomes calmer and some of the babies appear more able to relax into their mothers' arms. To complete the hour of music a goodbye song is sung, allowing the mothers and their babies to prepare to end today's group.

Conclusion

Playing music with mothers and their children helps to bring into focus the difficulties each couple may have, whilst facilitating a creative environment in which connections can be made and feelings expressed. It is essential that each mother feels she is accepted by the group as well as by the therapist. Mothers who are feeling bad about their babies as well as themselves may experience waves of guilt and in consequence can become frozen in their feelings. Sharing with others can enable a mother to 'come to life' for her baby and in consequence help her baby to begin to find a self which is accepted and has a place in the world.

Working with a group in a mainstream secondary school

Luke Annesley

This group has been running for four and a half years in a mainstream secondary school in London. The group members, on the whole, have a diagnosis of ASD and/or social/communication difficulties. From the outset my inclination was towards a low intervention, perhaps 'group analysis', type of approach. Musically this was about keeping in mind an ideal of group improvisation, with the emphasis on shared musical attention rather than, necessarily, musical coherence. There were times when I doubted the usefulness of this stance towards this particular group. I found myself wondering: would it be better to be more structured, even *much* more structured, and more firmly in the role of leader or 'group facilitator'? Would the music 'make more sense'? There were times in the group's early stages when I felt that nothing was happening, that the music in the session was so fragmented and the communication between the group members so sporadic that I wasn't sure whether the experience was really helping anyone. I think Foulkes' *conductor* role is what I aspired to. Perhaps this was a result of my training, including my own experience of being a member of an experiential training group. It may also be because I had experience running groups in a teaching role and I wanted to make a clear distinction in my own mind and my own practice between this and my new identity as a 'music therapist'.

Over time my own contribution to the group has become more robust. I think these early experiences of fragmentation and emptiness were valuable, but I have also come to believe that this particular group needs more holding, more encouragement towards interaction. There came a point about two years ago when one group member, Peter, suddenly announced that this was his final session, as from the following week he would be out of school on the day when the group took place. He did this as he was leaving the room at the end of the session, taking me by surprise. The group at this time had four members, plus the therapist, and he had been attending since the beginning. His leaving was a significant event for both him and the rest of us. My response was to negotiate for him to return for one more session, and this took several weeks to happen. In this final session Peter led the group in an improvisation which he held by playing a repeating chord sequence on guitar. There was a shared pulse, mutual musical awareness and a sense of group cohesiveness about this event. Everyone present was playing, and I was able to sit back and play the triangle quietly, enjoying this moment of shared music. Although Peter's ending process had been somewhat abrupt, perhaps it had 'woken me up' and forced me to become more proactive, not being swept along by the group, but taking charge a bit more in a helpful way.

One general tendency within the group is for people to drift off into their own separate musical worlds. One might be trying to play a learned tune on the keyboard while another plays an unrelated pulse, and another explores music apps on an iPad (a recent addition to the toolbox). In a recent session I intervened by stopping the group and drawing attention to the difficulty of the group being musically together. I suggested we try using the iPad together. The suggestion was ostensibly ignored, but the dynamic of the group shifted to a greater mutual awareness. More connected music ensued. This is a common experience, that my attempt to generate cohesion is brushed off, but then the group members find their own way. Another useful intervention when I have a trainee working with me in the group is for the two of us to lay down a groove together, modelling shared music and inviting others to join in. In another recent session this proved useful in addressing a particularly chaotic moment, enabling the therapists to assert their presence and allowing a couple of the group members to engage with our music.

One member, John, has been with the group since the beginning, and still is today, although he is soon to be leaving the school. His musical persona has at times been disruptive. He can sometimes sit at the piano, not playing, even closing his eyes and appearing to fall asleep. As I sometimes find that the piano is my best tool for providing musical coherence for the group, this can be frustrating. John has also gone through periods of sporadic attendance, but this has changed in the past year. He has become, through turnover of personnel, a senior group member, presiding over the new junior members from lower years. Part of the routine of our sessions centres on the djembe drum. We use this at the beginning and end of the session, with all of the group members sitting around the drum and finding an area of the drum's surface for themselves. However fragmented the rest of the session, there is cohesion at these times. John has recently become more active in encouraging this. He'll also turn to people at times if he's unhappy about what they're doing, saying 'You just killed it.'

John's longest period of non-attendance lasted for several weeks, and I was on the verge of admitting defeat. Messages had come to me via other members of staff and group members that John no longer wished to attend the group. It was my persistence in encouraging him, via other members of staff, and through chance encounters in the school corridor, to come along 'for at least one session' to discuss whether he wished to continue that finally led to his reappearance towards the end of a session. After this, his attendance pattern shifted. There was no more discussion about leaving, and he began to attend more regularly again. He began to try out different ways of being in the group, being more assertive with the other members. John became less a 'harbinger of doom' and more a 'guardian of the flame'. He became more likely to initiate shared drumming at the beginning and end, to suggest to other group members that they join in, on one occasion encouraging a wavering group member to stay to the end of a session.

One ingredient which has crept into the group over time and which I feel increasingly able to participate in is humour. There's a lot of joking around in the group and this is in some ways when it feels most alive. Having a sense of humour in therapy is perhaps not talked about much but I think it is part of what keeps this group going. John has again embodied this. The group takes him seriously, but not too seriously.

The group lives on and feels that it has a stronger identity now than at any other time in its short history. There have been more moments of musical cohesiveness than in the past. For John I think it has been an important presence. My role has shifted too, and perhaps this reflects something of John's experience. I have gone from beginner therapist, intervening very little, being little more than a presence in the group and a caretaker of the boundaries, to feeling involved as a real person, and at times an equal musical participant in shared interactions. It would seem that an important part of finding one's identity as a therapist is learning to bring more and more of a congruent persona into the sessions, while maintaining the right therapeutic stance. This is a continuing process and perhaps something that just can't be rushed.

Group music therapy with PTSD sufferers

Ann Sloboda and Catherine Carr

Introduction

This material is taken from a clinical trial conducted in 2008 which offered a period of ten weekly group music therapy sessions at the Guildhall School of Music and Drama to people suffering from post-traumatic stress disorder (PTSD) (Carr, d'Ardenne, Sloboda, Wang, Scott and Priebe 2012). PTSD is diagnosed when a person has either witnessed or been part of an event that they perceive as directly threatening to life and results in symptoms including dissociation, hyperarousal, emotional numbing and flashbacks of the event. PTSD has associated negative impacts on sufferers' everyday lives as they seek to avoid any experience that may trigger these symptoms; they may suffer depression and social isolation. All participants had completed recommended treatment from a local specialist centre providing psychological treatment for trauma, but had been discharged still experiencing severe symptoms of PTSD.

The rationale for offering group music therapy included practical factors such as resources available and that it resembled music therapy within NHS mental health settings. It was also significantly different from treatment participants had previously received.

The outcomes of this study were positive, with participants showing a significant reduction in symptoms at the end of therapy. The opportunity to work with such a homogenous group of patients is rare in ordinary clinical practice. Music therapy group techniques (Davies and Richards 2002) of employing loosely structured improvisation and verbal reflection proved effective in engaging the group and enabled participants to bring and work with specific trauma-related issues.

The group

The group consisted of three men and six women: Jacob (20), Mateo (20), Ivan (56), Alice (21), Isabella (32), Joanna (37), Claudia (40), Helen (30) and Maria (50). All had suffered multiple and sustained traumatic events including imprisonment, torture, bullying and sexual assault. Two members (Mateo and Helen) were British, whilst others came from countries in Eastern Europe, Africa and the Middle East. Five had asylum seeker status and some were uncertain if they would be able to remain in the UK or be returned to the country they had left. Some of the women in the group had ongoing problems with domestic violence and children who were born as a result of sexual assault. Three members had English as their first language and two were able to speak and understand English quite well, whilst the remaining four could only do so to a basic level. Participants were told briefly what to expect, but by and large had very little idea of what music therapy might involve.

Whilst the therapists had not worked exclusively with patients with a primary diagnosis of PTSD before, we set out to conduct the group using the same techniques that we would employ in an acute psychiatric setting. We anticipated that the anxiety of the group was likely to be heightened, given the unfamiliarity of all aspects of the experience and that therefore greater emphasis might need to be given to a supportive approach. We were also mindful that participants could experience dissociation or flashbacks during the sessions so were watchful for any signs of this. We agreed that Ann Sloboda (AS) would take the role of verbal leadership within the session and that Catherine Carr (CC) would take a supportive musical role, with the option of responding to individuals if necessary.

The first session

This began with structured musical activities led by the therapists, designed to reduce anxiety levels and to provide a gradual, staged introduction to the experience of free improvisation in a group. The first was an introductory activity of passing an instrument around, which each person would play on briefly and say his or her name. This activity was then extended to two instruments, so that members took turns to play a brief duet. AS then introduced the idea of the entire group improvising together. She first suggested that people choose an instrument that interested them and focus on their own sounds on that instrument. They were then encouraged to begin listening to other players around them and to try to link their sounds; initially with one other person, and then with others in the room.

The role of the piano was central to the early group experiences, as it provided a solid base, below the more rapid percussion beats played by the patients. The therapists' intention was to provide some coherence and to reduce the sense of anxiety or confusion, whilst avoiding imposing any restrictive rhythmic or melodic element that would impede members' freedom.

Whilst no specific instruction had been given to imitate each other, the more general suggestion of 'tuning into' at least one other person was largely taken up by imitating some aspect of each other's playing. The therapists' instruments had an important role in helping members to orientate themselves within the soundscape. Interestingly, some comments from the subsequent discussion formed the thematic basis of later group events. Members said they felt calmer after the improvisations and several expressed relief that they had been able to create some music as a group.

Some sounds had a strong effect on people. When commenting on the singing bowl, one person said 'that bell goes through my head!' whilst another commented 'I think it's an amazing instrument,' indicating the possibility of tension over conflicting instrumental preferences. The idea that emotions could be elicited and expressed on certain instruments was discussed, and some personal information was shared, with the idea that people might use the group for self-disclosure.

In reflection after the group, the therapists wondered if members might be fearful of joining in a common pulse and therefore remained rhythmically separate from one another, to preserve a sense of individuality. It was striking that, for most members, traumatic events had occurred in a context involving more than one person and this first encounter might have reminded them of prior destructive group experiences.

Subsequent sessions

The structural framework of the first session was used for subsequent sessions, with subtle variations. Its loose structure allowed spontaneous verbal or musical events to take place. The main shift over the weeks was an increased sense of autonomy, as members developed a greater capacity to make decisions and to participate with fewer directions from the therapists. Interpretations were kept to a minimum, the style being predominantly supportive and reflective.

Despite its loose and improvisatory nature, the sense of an overall structure and a general group culture helped to reduce anxiety and allow members to take risks within the session. Examples of risks included:

- getting up from a seat in the circle to go and play the piano;
- feeling safe enough to be less guarded and controlled or to play new instruments (the combination of this with active music making enabled an experience within a predictable structure where the participant could exert some control);
- being able to develop a vocabulary to acknowledge emotions;
- announcing dislike of the sound of a particular instrument and being able to relate this to traumatic experiences;
- admitting to feelings of anger and painful memories that came to mind whilst playing.

The penultimate session

The penultimate session was a pivotal point in the course of the therapy. Members were aware that only one more session was left and used this session to reflect upon their experiences within the group.

The session began with the passing around of temple blocks. Four members were present with the others unable to attend (family wedding; wife ill; new job; course). After the introductions, the group moved into an improvisation. Helen went immediately to the temple blocks which had previously been passed around. Joanna played the piano and later moved to the djembe; Isabella chose the djembe. AS and CC played piano and xylophone respectively, CC later moving to small percussion. Helen played very energetically and rhythmically and was completely absorbed in exploring the temple blocks in a very lively way. As this progressed, her facial expression changed from being relaxed to a frown and she became flushed, playing the instrument with more force. Alice arrived a couple of minutes into this improvisation and also played djembe. Alice and Joanna developed a shared unit rhythmically and instrumentally, both playing djembes and sharing the cymbal, taking turns freely. Jacob played guitar, strumming vigorously, and Helen moved to the piano. Partway through, AS stopped and moved to a drum, but did not play as the music felt it had momentum and energy of its own. The music was very synchronised and held together. No one drum dominated; each had its own equal part.

After this improvisation, several members began to speak of their experience in the group and the aspects of it that had been personally significant for them. AS commented that the music had been very energetic and that this had come from the participants. Alice said it was fun, although her tense body language did not match this. Jacob spoke about being in the middle and being surrounded by instruments – the music shutting out other thoughts and experiences. Joanna said she was almost dancing and commented that she often found herself 'drumming' on the bus after music therapy sessions. Isabella said she felt strong when drumming. Helen spoke of her worry that instruments might not be able to withstand the strength of playing and that she might break them. Helen reflected that when playing instruments in the group she really felt 'I can be me' when she usually feels as though she is above herself looking down. Other group members nodded at this statement. She said that this 'me' was herself before all the bad things had happened. Jacob commented that the group was a place where you could be safe from everything else. We wondered whether this perhaps implied internal safety as well as external. Joanna said that the group was something to look forward to on Fridays.

At the end of the session, the group was very quiet. AS said everybody had worked very hard in both playing and what they had said and that they had said some very important things. People were gaining support from the group. Helen said 'Everybody knows what you've been through.' As AS noted that it was time to finish, all sat quietly for a minute and none seemed ready to leave immediately.

The anti-group and the experiential group

Alison Davies

Building on the thoughts about the anti-group in Chapter 7 of this book, this is an example of an anti-group dynamic played out in the early stages of a music therapy experiential group.

A group of students starting their music therapy training spent the first two weeks being very negative about the group. It was clear that the general feeling amongst members was that a group of this kind was 'artificial': wouldn't it be better to have a conversation over coffee or in the pub rather than endure the long silences that were happening? One group member suggested that the group improvise music together. As conductor, I thought this could be one way for the group to begin to feel together and connected in this strange alien group environment that they were experiencing, especially as it came from the group members themselves. Because the group had only met twice, members had not yet built up a sense of cohesion. Relationships with one another in the group were only beginning to be formed. Playing music might help a sense of being together. However, no one confronted or questioned the person who wanted the coffee or pub group and no one engaged with the suggestion about improvising music.

After a long silence one member, clearly desperate for something to happen, suggested that they all get up and dance a Samba around the room. A look of 'dare we?' came over the group; I was a bit taken aback, but I waited to see what would happen.

Group members began to dance a Samba in a circle around the room. I remained seated. After finishing dancing they sat in various places around the room abandoning the circle of chairs set out for the group. What followed was a discussion about how they had felt more in control when initiating their own dance than when being invited to improvise music together. I pointed to the anxiety that was present earlier in the group and suggested that maybe by dancing the Samba altogether they had arrived at their own sense of connecting to each other and being together. However, the structure of the dance, which was familiar to them all from a workshop that they had attended earlier in the day, was in my view a way of defending against the anxiety of the unknown. They were making every effort to make the experiential group like another task-orientated group or even a pub or coffee group. They then might feel they knew where they stood and what was expected of them.

Although I felt initially threatened by this anti-group display, some positive thinking came out of it. The group was able to look at how some feared not going along with the suggestion of the strong member of the group who initiated the idea of the dance but had also been anxious about what I, the conductor, might think. Some felt they were torn between remaining anxious in the group, waiting to see what might unfold, and wanting to do something together that they all knew. Others felt they wanted to do something that was at one level a bit defiant but at a deeper level was a challenge to what they saw as the conductor's authority and sense of control.

Initially what seemed like 'acting out' by group members dancing outside the group circle and forming into an anti-group proved to generate thought about the nature of anxiety and in particular about the nature of their anxiety about this group. From reflections on the known agenda of the Samba, group members were able to think about how hard it was to stay with the unknown element that the group presented them with. What had at the time seemed an anti-group presentation led to a lively discussion about the nature of being open to new experience.

Group cognitive analytic music therapy in a high secure hospital setting

Stella Compton Dickinson

Duggan et al. (2009) state that patients in secure hospital treatment who have restricted freedom and choice have a right to expect evidence-based treatments. There is therefore a need to evaluate the clinical effectiveness of forensic music therapy. This vignette will summarise how and why the principles of S.H. Foulkes are integrated into a context-specific model of forensic music therapy called cognitive analytic music therapy (CAMT) (Compton Dickinson 2006).

Foulkes (1948) regarded the social functioning of groups as basic to human existence. We are all born into groups, belonging to a greater or lesser degree to family, cultures and society. Through these influences the individual's life may be shaped both consciously and unconsciously; life within the culture of the therapy group may help to reshape the individual. Such a group may be a microcosm which reflects the culture of the wider organisation and society within which the group functions. Descriptive examples will be given from a pilot group in a high secure hospital.

Roberts (2013) highlights the group work treatment challenges of S.H. Foulkes' model with patients who are incarcerated and removed from mainstream society. She recognises the difficulties for these patients in developing intimacy due to their highly disturbed attachment patterns.

There are different social norms within the community of a high secure hospital and this presents challenges in the treatment aims of recovery and normalisation. It is a challenge to achieve a cohesive and functional group with severely mentally ill patients who have frequently suffered very abusive childhood experiences and who have impaired relating strategies as a result. Within the confines of a high secure hospital patients are constantly monitored. Security procedures and risk management are priorities. Anxiety levels are high in staff whose purpose is to maintain a functional, controlled, yet caring environment.

Foulkes suggests that 'the deepest reason why group analytic patients can reinforce each other's normal reactions and wear down and correct each other's neurotic reactions is that collectively they constitute the very norm from which, individually, they deviate' (1948). In forensic treatment, however, the patient 'norm' may be viewed as different from the external norm. These patients are already stigmatised as a danger to society, since they have already deviated from the social norm by committing a violent offence.

The treatment challenge is the 'index' offence for which each individual is committed to a secure hospital. This can become the elephant in the therapy room, since there is an unwritten rule that between themselves and on the wards patients are not encouraged to discuss their offences as this can lead to victimisation. Therefore, a strange sort of 'normalisation' occurs for the safety of the ward community and the individual. The music therapist must create a different sort of safe therapeutic environment where patients feel able to 'work' on why they are in treatment. This therapeutic process almost always involves the re-avowing of dissociated feelings which carries with it the risk of violent acting out.

Emotional expression through musical interaction, rather than with words, can be particularly useful with this patient group in facilitating the internal process of change. In this way the feeling behind the intentionality of behavioural response may be recognised and safely expressed by the patient, the therapist and the group as a whole. The explicit recognition of the underlying emotions of patients who have committed violent offences requires sensitive naming by the therapist at an appropriately timed moment. The patient's ability to see his own darker side otherwise remains impaired, and the reason why he is incarcerated, his index offence, with the accompanying negative and toxic emotions, remains untreated or may even be exacerbated.

Sleight and Compton (2013) describe this process in which 'Craig' recalled school and family memories of exclusion. These were reflected in how Craig was unable to integrate with the group's music making, and how this led to recognition and expression of anger at his experience of an emotionally blunted childhood. Craig then discovered he could find a musical outlet for this feeling, with threatening use of the claves (two hardwood sticks) hit together in a gradually intensified and increasingly fast rhythm which had a tribal effect on gathering the group into a potentially dangerous gang. This was so powerful that it led to a group 'war' which had to be contained and mediated by the two music therapists working together to avoid scapegoating, which Craig himself had suffered as a teenager (Sleight and Compton 2013). When repressed or dissociated feelings are positively and safely re-avowed this can amount to the expression of authentic feeling, a reduction of denial of the 'offender' state of being, and the possibility of feelings of remorse.

There are similarities between Foulkes' thinking and cognitive analytic therapy (CAT) (Ryle and Kerr 2002); these may be seen clearly within non-verbal and musical group interactions and transferences in cognitive analytic music therapy. Craig progressed to becoming able to recognise how excluded he had always felt and through reciprocal relating within this group model, in which dialogue is actively encouraged through jointly created music, he gained acceptance of himself by others and subsequently of himself. He could then address pre-disposing offence-related factors, which included many past humiliating experiences. His severely impaired social skills were ameliorated through the group's musical interaction.

This example demonstrates how the application of Foulkes' principles in cognitive analytic music therapy can throw light on complex issues by enabling clinicians to see the parallel processes linked to offence-related behaviours which re-occur and which can be ameliorated within the microcosm of the group. In CAT terminology, relating patterns are conceptualised and can be named to the group as 'reciprocal roles' (examples might be the ignoring self to the ignored other, or a rejecting other to a rejected self). Such reciprocal roles may be observed during musical interactions. In the CAT model, however, these roles are named rather than interpreted. Blunden (2010) explains how such responses and behaviours contribute to an internalised group dynamic.

The model provides cognitive and analytic understanding of how patients' impulses, projections and responses may be reflected in multi-disciplinary team dynamics, and at a higher level in organisational anxieties that manifest within the hierarchy of the high secure hospital system. For example, a patient may express feeling 'frustrated and confused' and the therapist in clinical supervision may express these same feelings.

Gahir and Compton (2013) describe joint work between a music therapist and a psychologist who had separate remits to work concurrently with a long-term, treatment-resistant patient, 'Ewan'. He presented with strong Oedipal tendencies; he had grown up witnessing parental conflict and domestic violence. The music therapist and the psychologist had to be seen by Ewan to support each other, or he would attempt to create a split, making one of them the good maternal part object, the other the bad paternal part object. Close liaison was required and the consultant psychiatrist held a parental function for the team. He contained the anxieties and the potential parallel splits between the therapist and the psychologist by facilitating meetings to discuss and resolve potential conflicts and different perspectives.

In sessions, patients are able to move freely around the music therapy room, rather than remaining seated. Destructive behaviours may be triggered through memories and feelings, which are elicited in the jointly created music. Responses of group members can feel problematic to the music therapist, such as a quiet member; an anxiously talkative member; a member who acts as though he is the group leader; a member who deflects everything away from himself and onto other members; or a member who relates everything to himself. The therapist therefore has to dance between attending to individual needs and to the group as a whole.

When Ewan progressed from individual to group cognitive analytic music therapy, a conflict emerged between him and a peer from the same ward. Envy and a transferential sibling rivalry developed in which Ewan, the more dominant patient, sought all the attention from the therapists. The weaker patient, significantly the only member of the group who had not killed, strove to take the role of peacemaker at all costs. This was a familiar position, which he had always taken in his biological family. Through the therapeutic process he discovered how to assert himself and to resolve conflict rather than to placate, and Ewan discovered how to share the space in greater harmony. This required energetic and conscious strategies of group containment and a developed co-working partnership between the two music therapists, through which they could facilitate balanced, aesthetically pleasing and mood-appropriate jointly created group music and a shared reciprocity which was ultimately reflected in the group members' responses.

In this way, the dialogical approach of G-CAMT contains and intentionally limits the free-floating narrative of group analysis. The aim is that through this group work process in which members may form closer bonds through carefully mediated, jointly created music each individual may discover a greater degree of interpersonal effectiveness and social feeling.

All groups offer members the chance to see something of themselves as others see them. This can be helpful or, at other times, painful and unnerving. In therapeutic group work with men who have committed serious offences, the impact of the index offence is primarily on the ability to self-reflect; to think about how they inflicted pain and/or death is not usually the explicit purpose of the music therapy group, but it is ignored at one's peril. The intra-psychic processes, much of which are unspeakable and may remain implicit, can however be expressed non-verbally in musical material which is then articulated verbally. This can lead to a re-connection with feelings and an ability to recognise behaviours, which may be dysfunctional and anti-social or helpful and constructive.

It was Craig who became the voice for the whole group in recognising and naming his feeling of being 'sad' when the group was preparing to end. This sadness in the present linked to his remorse for past actions and a more integrated and balanced emotional response. This newly recognised emotion demonstrated the value of group analytic principles as well as the flexibility and ongoing usefulness of integrating this model with cognitive analytic music therapy to create a context-specific, clinically effective intervention within the constraints of a time-limited within multi-disciplinary forensic treatment.

Making connections in a group for people with learning disabilities

Eleanor Richards

Dave, Colin, Teresa and Simon were four adults with moderate learning disabilities; they were members of a music therapy group which had been established for two years at the time of the events discussed here. Dave and Teresa were in the group from its inception; Colin and Simon joined a year later. Dave and Teresa lived near one another and sometimes met outside the group at a local day centre. The group worked through both improvised music and talking. All the group members were originally referred because they were thought to be having difficulties with social interaction; although they were in their late thirties, all still lived with their parents, and their day-to-day living was characterised by regular routines and rather limited engagement with the wider world. Their parents were ageing, and all group members were facing the possibility of loss and significant changes in their living arrangements in the coming years. The theme of death often came up in the group, usually indirectly through discussion of the experiences of their friends, or of events in the news. The vulnerability of the people being talked about was often emphasised. I think it felt important at that stage for the group to talk about other people; that enabled them to project some of their own sharpest fears into situations elsewhere, and to feel some kind of authority in being able to discuss others and show their knowledge.

Dave had Down's Syndrome; he was the person who had most difficulties with verbal interaction, as both his comprehension and his speech were at an early developmental stage. His parents were committed members of a church congregation, where he was much liked. He brought to the group the expectation that people would understand his speech and that even if they did not, they would make an effort to find out what he wanted. Taking his place in a group on equal terms was a struggle for him; he found it hard to witness verbal exchanges going on between other group members (particularly if Teresa was involved) which he could not always fully understand. He would react to such situations by attacking them in different ways; he might yawn exaggeratedly, or try to distract one of the speakers by making faces or in some other way being the clown. Perhaps because he and she knew one another outside the group, he would sometimes half jokingly try to imply a romantic connection with Teresa; she rejected those moves, but also giggled with some enjoyment.

Teresa was much more apparently verbally competent, and sought to sound as assured as she could. She used rather sophisticated language, but it was not always certain that she knew what her words meant; her need to present a functioning, independent self disguised her real difficulties with flexible, open conversation. Her music seemed at first rather competent, too; she found ways to play some percussion instruments that were quite skilled, but ultimately unchanging. She would get into a repetitive rhythm, which was useful for the group's music as a whole because of its steadiness, but which she held to doggedly, whatever else was happening in the music, playing with her head down, and not always immediately aware if other group members stopped playing. Dave, by contrast, could be flexible in the music in ways which were much more available to him than in verbal exchanges. He enjoyed devising sharp, edgy rhythms, and would actively look round the group for someone to have a dialogue with. He was also attuned to mood, and could equally take part in more thoughtful, slow moving music. Sometimes he would take the safe option of following someone else (usually the conductor), but often he would find a means with confidence to try to take the music in a new direction by changing the sound or volume of his playing. He clearly enjoyed not only the music but the place his part in it gave him in the group, which contrasted so sharply with his experience of verbal exchange. Colin and Simon tended to take roles that put them more in the background, listening and responding but rarely taking initiatives.

Gradually, however, Simon began to show some irritation with Dave's clowning attempts to disrupt conversations; Dave responded by withdrawing his attention and looking out of the window, or by making a long visit to the toilet, and once or twice he made a half mocking threatening gesture towards Simon with a beater.

Teresa arrived at one session with some difficult family news: her uncle had been killed in a road accident. She started to talk about it with the rather calm, detached tone that she often brought to conversations, but gradually found herself distraught and tearful. Simon and Colin were at a loss; her grief exposed their difficulty in resonating with another's feelings. Simon responded with rather stilted phrases, and Colin was silent and anxious.

I am not sure that Dave understood what had happened, but he watched intently as Teresa spoke and others responded, and did not try to disrupt the situation with jokes. Instead, he got Colin to change places with him so that he could sit next to Teresa, and began to play a slow, careful tune on the bass metallophone. I supported it occasionally on the piano. After a while Dave handed Teresa a beater so that she could play a large drum that was in front of her. She joined in with us and her playing gradually became stronger, so that at the climax of the piece she was playing loud, steady drumbeats with real physical engagement, which seemed to voice the depth of her grief and anger. Gradually the other two joined in, and the whole group made an ending to the music together. Teresa breathed out slowly, and we sat in silence.

Dave's intuitive response to Teresa's state of mind found its expression in music in a way that he could not have conveyed in words, and which freed Teresa from the need to respond with her own apparently more competent, but stilted verbal resources. Colin and Simon were also able to take part in the group's shared voicing of the feeling in the room.

The appearance of this music, more focused and expressive than anything the group had found together before, was in itself striking. Even more importantly, it was part of a continuing group process. Dave had found some emotional authority which allowed him thereafter to be more calmly attentive to group events with less need for envious disruptions. Teresa's playing became more flexible and she responded more readily to the changes in the music.

People with learning disabilities may have difficulty in articulating their experience in words, but may nonetheless be, often for defensive reasons, very watchful and emotionally perceptive. Working through improvised music allows that perceptiveness to be articulated and exchanged and to serve more positive purposes; it may also allow group members to feel more readily that their experience is recognised and echoed.

Chapter 12

Co-therapy and working with others

Alison Davies

Introduction

This chapter looks at aspects of working with others in a music therapy setting. I will explore various dynamics: where both therapists are of equal status as music therapists; when one is a music therapist and the other or others are from different professional disciplines; when a trained music therapist is working with a trainee; when two music therapy students are working together; and where assistants are present in sessions in order to support the needs of particular clients.

It is often argued that to have more than one therapist for a group is not cost effective. Fewer institutions nowadays have more than one music therapist, whereas in the 1970s to 1990s it was more common for an arts therapies department to employ several. It is still worth considering the dynamics of the co-therapy relationship, however, and the valuable insights that this way of working can bring.

Foulkes, group analysis and co-therapy

The group analyst Inge Hudson (2008) looks at how S.H. Foulkes viewed co-therapy and suggests that it is often considered that he thought little about co-therapy and did not really consider it in any depth. It has little prominence in his writing and consequently has scarcely been written about amongst group analysts. She draws attention to the only passage in Foulkes' writing that mentions co-therapy. In 'The Conductor in Action' (1975a/1986) he says

> A word may be said here about having a co-conductor sitting in. This is of great value for teaching purposes and has certain advantages. On the whole it is my observation that the group itself is better off with one conductor. At any rate one should be in charge, and the other more of an assistant conductor. This second conductor may at times take over and he can make a very valuable contribution and need in no way be given second rank.
>
> Foulkes (1975a/1986: 105)

Foulkes' idea that a co-therapist should be an assistant is rather contradicted by his subsequent comment. Despite this approach, co-therapy relationships can be considered a good model in group therapy, where relationships are at the heart of the process. Hudson also points to an interesting comment from family therapy literature:

> It is no accident that co-therapy has been from the beginning an important technique in family therapy – for it introduces into the treatment situation a therapeutic **relationship** instead of simply a therapeutic **individual.** This is clearly appropriate in the context of a treatment modality whose focus is the interrelationship between individuals rather than the individuals themselves ... The relationship between the workers becomes more than just simply the sum of its parts. It is, in itself, a dynamic entity, which, more than the treatment interventions of either partner alone, holds the germ of truth and change for the family.
>
> Walrond-Skinner (1976: 110–11)

She notices how close this relational approach is to that of group analysis and concludes that co-therapy could be a very natural model to consider in relation to groups.

Why work with others?

Depending on the resources available, the culture of the institution and the type and size of the group, it can be a matter of preference whether to work alone or with others. Some music therapists value the support of another therapist to witness with them the dynamics of the group, and its struggles and process. In a good co-therapy relationship, partners will be open to each other's approaches and learn from one other. As well as the wisdom that a more senior therapist might offer, there is also value in what the less experienced therapist may bring in terms of fresh thoughts.

Managing the needs of certain client groups such as a children's group, or a group of people with disabilities, may necessitate other people being in the room. Whether or not they are considered co-therapists, all in the room are part of the dynamics of the group.

Two co-therapists are often seen by the group as the parental couple. Behr and Hearst (2005) write:

> the very fact that there is a 'couple' influences the dynamics of the group. As well as being experienced as the parental couple, they may be seen as sexual partners, and fantasies will arise, and will need to surface in the session, about their lives outside the group, especially during breaks in the therapy. Group fantasies exert a strong unconscious power on the therapists, who

may find themselves acting out some of the attributes assigned to them by the group.

Behr and Hurst (2005: 34–35)

Where the group perceives a parental couple, that can model both the fact that two parents can get on and live relatively harmoniously, and also that they can have differences and not fall out. This might be especially useful to observe for group members who have experienced parents in conflict.

Two music therapists working together

In a paper in the *British Journal of Music Therapy* in 1998, Eleanor Richards and I discussed co-therapy work with an open group in an acute psychiatric setting.

The context

We decided to run a joint music therapy group offering it to two acute admission wards in the same building. The patients on these wards had a variety of problems. For some this was their first admission; for others it might be one among repeated admissions, perhaps when a more chronic condition was undergoing an acute phase. Diagnoses varied from neurotic symptoms – anxiety, depression, stress – to more psychotic presentations such as manic depression or schizophrenia. The group was open to anyone on the ward who wished to come. So in principle we were an open group for the ward – open to all sorts of unexpected happenings (Davies and Richards 1998: 54).

How we saw our roles

> It seems unusual, in this country at least, for two qualified music therapists to work together as co-therapists. Both of us have experience of working together as co-therapists with other professionals who are non-musicians, but working together altered the function of the music in the group, and certainly differently informed the nature of the working relationship between the therapists. For both of us this had been our first substantial experience of working with another music therapist since our respective trainings.
>
> At the start we knew very little of one another's musical 'personalities' or predispositions, and part of the process of developing together has been the ongoing investigation of our musical relationship. Like any other aspect of a co-working relationship this has not always been an easy area. Has one found the other too dominant or reticent? Is my music appropriate? How can we best address issues – in the review or in supervision? Broadly, the ways in which we have functioned musically can be thought of in relation to our other non-musical roles in the group. Most usually one of us has played the

142 Clinical perspectives

piano: we have thought of that role within the music as one of containing, in that it can provide a resonant framework of sound within which a network of events and interactions can take place, and in its own music seek to reflect something of the group mind. The other therapist remains available to engage with or support individual members or a distinctive strand within the music, to be involved with the playing on a practical level (assisting people with instruments if necessary) and to observe visually more of the events of the group . . . Most importantly, we have sought to be flexible in our sharing of these fundamental activities and to move readily between them as the session proceeds.

Davies and Richards (1998: 56–7)

A dynamic that emerged between us

There have been times when it has been essential for our development as a partnership to acknowledge areas of difficulty and discuss them. A useful example here is an instance in which it seemed that one of us was doing most of the talking. Both of us were aware of the imbalance, but it was in supervision that we were first able to address it clearly. Perhaps one of us was feeling anxious that the group might somehow fall apart, and the responsibility for making sure things 'happened' in the group, whilst the other therapist was more prepared to wait and was in any case feeling that there was little space to speak. Both of us were feeling some anger – or at least discomfort – and it was during and after supervision in which this dynamic was a central issue that we were both able to express our feelings more directly and, equally importantly, to look at how such a situation had arisen, not least by closely examining events in the clinical setting.

That particular instance arose in the context of our respective responses to a group member. L was a woman who, in several sessions, dominated the group, talking a great deal. She spoke angrily yet somehow superficially of her feelings and circumstances. She said repeatedly that she must find a 'solution' for things herself, but at the same time made it clear that there were limits to what she was prepared to do or risk in the group and that for her, probably change could never happen. She added to this implicit attack on the group process and, by extension, the therapists, by repeating in various ways her mistrust of the music, often in quite contemptuous terms. Her involvement in playing was half-hearted or tentative and she belittled the group's music (and thus others' engagement) by talking about it as 'just noise' or, rather academically as 'three separate strands'.

We, the therapists, became polarised. A's (Alison's) response, perhaps taking on some of L's underlying desperation, was to respond to her with some of the same urgency and with a lot of words, seizing opportunities to make connections or suggestions, and often being told by L that she had got it wrong. As A took on some of L's desire to think, or her illusions of thought, with its inherent frustration and rising anxiety, but constant impulse to verbalise and fill up space, so E found herself feeling things which seemed related to other aspects of L's experience and also to the experience of other members of the group. E found it difficult to think or respond creatively; she was much more silent and perhaps took on some of the feelings of the rest of the group of apparent paralysis – and resentment – in the face of so much verbal material. A wished E was saying more – as on some level L wanted more from the group, whilst at the same time excluding them; E felt that there was no space, either in her head or in the room, to respond.

Both of us felt very conscious of the difficulty and referred to it occasionally, but it was in supervision that we were able to be most open, both about our respective feelings and about what seemed to be going on in the group. This was a valuable moment, not least because it moved us forward in our relationship as co-therapists.

Davies and Richards (1998: 58)

Supervision helped us to see that the dynamic that we were experiencing between us as co-therapists in the group could be considered a mirror image of the dynamics with which the group was struggling. Awareness of our own interactions with each other and in our roles as therapists allowed us to be much more available for the group members as we were no longer stuck in a difficult unaddressed co-therapy relationship. Understanding what was happening between us and seeing how it paralleled the dynamics of the group was an important turning point in our co-therapy relationship. For myself, I could see more clearly how I had become caught up in the anxiety of the group, expressed by this particular over-anxious individual group member, generating my desire to try and make something happen.

Musically, two music therapists have the advantage of different roles in the group. One can support the music of the group, for instance on the piano or by the use of a rhythmic drum beat, whilst the other can be more aware of the overall group process. Both therapists will be listening to what is played, but one can be more musically active than the other. The more interactive therapist will be tuning into the mood of the music whilst the other might be tuning into what is happening non-musically, for instance with a group member who does not play or has a disruptive attitude that indicates difficulty in joining in or being together.

Co-therapy with a qualified music therapist and trainee

This is a situation where a trainee music therapist has the opportunity to work in a music therapy group with an experienced music therapist. This has good learning potential but also brings difficulties that need to be thought through.

Firstly, the setting is relatively safe and protected for the trainee music therapist who can learn from someone more experienced. Sometimes the trainee looks forward to that; at other times it might be rather daunting. The trainee's 'authority' in the group may feel unclear and group members may feel ambivalent towards her. Is she 'one of us' or not? The trainee has to conduct herself with authority in spite of her relatively limited experience.

The trainee may feel inhibited about trying interventions, verbal or musical, because she fears being judged. This can be an issue for both therapists, but for the trainee this is a very real anxiety; a report on her work may have to be prepared at the end of the placement. However, the role of the experienced music therapist is to help and encourage the trainee to take risks, to get it wrong sometimes, and to learn from the experience. Good communication between the two needs to be established so that each can be clear with the other as to what their roles are.

For the established music therapist, the added dynamic of having a trainee as a co-therapist can feel quite a responsibility. As well as having to consider her own transference and countertransference, she has the added presence of a trainee and all that this brings. At the same time, as the more experienced therapist, she has to take care of the group and provide a therapeutic environment for the group members. She therefore has a dual role. Like the trainee, she may also feel under scrutiny. Am I giving this trainee a good enough experience? Do I really know what I am doing? Can I stay in the realm of 'not knowing' and still be useful to the trainee? And what might get reported back about my work to the training institution? In various ways, both therapists may feel under pressure.

The dynamics that arise between trained music therapist, trainee and the group members can be thought about fruitfully in supervision. What happens in the group between the therapists will inevitably be reflected in the dynamics of the group. That is where outside supervision can be invaluable, but also may have to be sensitively conducted if one therapist is a trainee. In a situation where a trainee is a co-therapist, discussion and debriefing are available after the session, but the trainee takes her work back to college for supervision, where she can have a space to voice doubts and anxieties that she might not find easy to express in front of her co-therapist. One institution, however, arranged a separate supervisory meeting just to look at co-therapy dynamics where a trainee and qualified music therapist were working together. This allowed both therapists to share with a supervisor their experiences and anxieties from their different perspectives. The student then took her work in the group back to be supervised by her training organisation.

Two student trainee music therapists

It is quite common for students to work together as co-therapists in a music therapy group whilst training. Many of the issues considered in this chapter arise in a student co-partnership; the added dynamic of training together may heighten anxieties and competition. Students may have different musical strengths; if any competitiveness that arises is not spoken about, it can get in the way of working together. In music therapy groups where there is verbal exchange as well as music, the ability to hold one's own in both these modalities can vary greatly. Discussing with one another where their individual strengths and weaknesses lie can be a very enabling and mature step to take; students can then learn by watching and taking in from each other. They may have to accept the idea that this is the time to make mistakes and learn from them, even if it is in front of peers. In this respect they may discover they have more to offer each other than they had thought at the outset. The comfort of not being alone in one's first ventures with groups can be reassuring.

Supervision, as always, is important, and especially so for students. A supervisor, one step removed from the clinical situation, can be helpful, as in previous examples, in looking at how the dynamics of the co-therapy relationship may resonate with aspects of the group being supervised. With sensitive and supportive supervision, discovering these dynamics can be exciting and may deepen the work.

An example

Two students who are working together as co-therapists have different backgrounds that have led them to train as music therapists. S has recently graduated from music college, is a very able violinist, and can also improvise freely on the piano. F, her co-therapist, is an older woman who has worked as a teacher and been a student counsellor. Her musical skills are good but she is acutely aware that she does not have S's spontaneous ability to improvise. Each is nervous about working with the other. S, in her anxiety, takes every opportunity to go to the piano and provide a strong harmonic and rhythmic base. She will often initiate music before group members do. F holds back, often thinking that the group needs to be eased into the music by talking with each other. This dynamic is around for some time, with S and F feeling that they cannot talk to each other about it because it would expose their weaknesses. However, in supervision they are gradually able to look at this dynamic between them when it is pointed out that the same problem is manifesting itself in the group.

One group member said they could not play an instrument, especially in front of others. Another said that they always felt inadequate if they could not do what others are able to. Someone else in the group dismissed the musical side as being 'childish', whilst another seemed painfully shy when it came to the talking but could 'shine', as she put it, when they played music.

Both therapists became aware through supervision that the group members' dilemmas had similarities with how they, as co-therapists, felt about each other. By working on their co-therapy relationship, acknowledging their individual skills, each became able to value the contribution of the other. The idea that there was enough to go round, and that if one person had certain skills maybe the other person could also gain them, helped them free up and become more relaxed and so more open to learning from each other. Through that they were also gaining insight into what might be going on for group members. They could then make empathic connections in the group as they saw the group struggling in the same way they were themselves.

Co-therapists from different disciplines

Particular dynamics may arise in a group when the therapy partners are from different disciplines. In a psychiatric setting, for instance, a nurse, occupational therapist or psychologist might ask to join the group run by a music therapist. They may then have the opportunity of encountering aspects of a patient that they may not have observed in another context.

Music therapy in a group with elderly people, for example, can often enliven and motivate group members who otherwise might remain passive, isolated and cut off from others. This potentially more engaged side of the patient is good for staff to see and may serve to energise their approach to the patients outside the group.

Mutual respect for each other's disciplines is all-important here, and joint supervision is the best place to look at issues that may be under the surface and causing the co-working relationship to be problematic. Music therapists and other professionals have much to offer each other and co-working in a group can lead to a creative interchange in the service of the wellbeing of the patients.

Hudson points to the importance of '... not trying to deny the differences between the therapists, because the group can work this out anyway, but to work towards a state of affairs where both therapists are perhaps taking somewhat different but complementary and equally valuable roles' (2008: 7).

Helpers in a group

Helpers in the form of care or teaching assistants are sometimes included in a music therapy group. It is important to recognise that whoever is in the room, even in the capacity of helper, contributes to the dynamics. This may be challenging for the music therapist depending on the level of awareness that the helper brings to the music therapy process. Meeting with helpers, explaining to them the nature of music therapy and what their role as helpers or assistants might be in the group, is important. They may know their particular patient well from outside the group, but very often they can see new sides through observing their participation in the music. Mutual respect again for the role helpers and assistants play in the lives of their patients is important and a sensitive approach on the part of the music therapist can significantly help them take an appropriate place in the group.

Pitfalls do occur and the most common one is for helpers or nurses to indulge in thinking the group is for their own and not the patients' needs. This is rarely conscious and might be a reaction to suddenly being in a group with music where the idea of self-expression is unfamiliar to them and at some level they 'want to have a go' too. Often the idea of music therapy is so new to helpers that they need guidance as to how to be in the group.

A group within the group

The dynamics that transpire in a group led by two therapists or multiple leaders form in effect a double process. As Levine and Dang (1979) point out, the co-therapists make up an inner group that has its own process to work through whilst at the same time facilitating the process of the group they are conducting. Any unresolved issues pertaining to the co-therapy dyad or co-worker combination may be reflected in the therapy group itself. Just as the patient therapy group has to work through unconscious resistances, so the co-therapists may have to look at unconscious issues that may have potential to cause an impasse if they are not explored. Supervision is the best place to address this.

Supervision

It is most helpful when the therapists in a co-therapy relationship attend supervision together. 'Since the group of leaders is without its own therapist, . . . supervision plays an important role in assisting the co-therapy team to identify and resolve its difficulties' (Levine and Dang 1979: 175).

Hudson (2008) draws attention to aspects of co-therapy that the therapy couple may be unaware of. 'Supervision helps to identify blind spots, thus guarding against acting out of something that has been projected into the co-therapy couple by the group.'

One dynamic that may be useful to address in supervision is the idea that the co-therapy couple, irrespective of gender, can play out masculine and feminine roles. This in turn may reflect the parental couple. Co-therapists of the same sex can equally have masculine and feminine roles assigned to them by group members.

Eleanor Richards and I wrote this about our joint supervision:

> Supervision has been very important. One element we have found helpful is the idea of the parental couple represented by the co-therapists. By this we mean what we have come to call the masculine and feminine elements or the feminine 'container' element and the masculine 'organising' component. We have found it useful to recognise these roles in our partnership and to be able to move between them. We would consider the feminine role, the container, to be closer to that of the nurturer, perhaps the one who looks for underlying feelings, and the masculine role to be more interpretative and managing. We thought it important to recognise when we might, as co-therapists get stuck in these roles. Sometimes co-therapy relationships can founder because the 'stuckness' is not recognised and there is envy or over-valuing of either the more penetrative, clever, interpretative role,

or of the ability to uncover feelings and provide a nurturing atmosphere. We found that in supervision when these elements were honestly and openly discussed we could move freely between the two roles, and felt that we (each) could develop both so-called masculine and feminine attributes in ourselves.

Davies and Richards (1998: 57–58)

Some final thoughts

One consideration from a practical point of view is that the employment of two therapists allows the group to have the potential to continue when one therapist is unavoidably absent or when one therapist has to leave the group permanently. Useful material might come up in the group if that happens. Themes of loss and abandonment come to mind, and can be explored with the therapist present.

Concerning possible transference on to co-therapists, McGee and Schuman (1970) write:

> With respect to dynamic considerations, the following concepts can be put forward. The great majority of individuals have had two major transferences in their lives, i.e., a mother and a father. Generally speaking, they have had to share these transference objects with siblings. In a certain sense, a group conducted by co-therapists comes closer to replicating the original family constellation than does the group operated by only one therapist. The use of co-therapists enriches the range and type of possible transference objects among group members and therapists. Also, with the presence of a co-therapist, additional facets of each therapist's personality are available for scrutiny by group members.
>
> McGee and Schuman (1970: 26)

For a music therapist it is always of prime interest to be aware of the dynamics taking place in the music. Observations in the music by two or more therapists can add to the insights of the whole group. The therapists' different senses of group members' music may also be valuable in providing alternative perspectives. Feelings arising from the loss of a therapist or group member can not only be articulated in words by the therapists, but played and felt through the music by the whole group.

Co-therapy and co-working can be very fruitful ways of working together; the presence and thinking of others within the same process can have many benefits.

Chapter 13

Experiential groups on music therapy trainings

Alison Davies

In all music therapy trainings in the UK a student experiential group is a key element in the training process. Here I will discuss the nature of this type of group when it uses the modalities of both words and music, looking through a group analytic lens at how that may enhance understanding of the group process and provide an integral part of the learning and personal growth of a music therapist in training. The technical terms referred to are an expansion in terms of music therapy of theory that is discussed elsewhere in this book by Nick Barwick.

The journey

A boat is preparing to leave the harbour. It pulls up anchor and is on its way. For the early part of the journey, voyagers can still see the land from which they set sail. There is a desire for exploration towards the future but an equal anxiety about leaving the safety of the land. However, there comes a point at which, out in mid-ocean, those on board can see neither the harbour from which they set sail nor the land ahead. The sea may be rough and anxieties great amongst the crew. Each member is dependent on the other. Each has a responsibility for the other as well as for themselves. Risks may have to be taken but they are all in this together. Finally, the destination comes into view and the boat is steered towards the harbour where each person will go their own way, taking with them the experience of their journey together. This may be 'terra firma' but there is also an accompanying loss of the many aspects of being with each other that has bound them together.

The context of the group

An experiential group for trainees can thus be looked on as a journey. Students all begin the group together and mostly end together. They share the main goal of training – to become music therapists – and, to varying degrees, have musical expertise in common. Usually the group is mixed in terms of age, gender, nationality and life experience. Though the group may take place in the same premises as the students' study environment, it nevertheless hopes to offer students a very particular kind of space, different from that encountered on the rest of the course. Within this space, tuned and un-tuned musical instruments are available to play. These are usually but not always placed centrally in the room, surrounded by a circle of chairs. Students are also encouraged to bring their own personal instruments.

Experiential groups on music therapy trainings are not stranger groups. Group members meet outside the group on the music therapy study programme. Indeed, they see one another in a variety of contexts and are witness to each other's abilities, expertise and differences in study activities, both academic and musical. These shared experiences of training are often pertinent to, and played out in, the dynamic material that subsequently evolves in the experiential group. More homogeneous than a therapy group, the experiential group is time limited and closed.

What is the group for?

Although there is no structure or agenda, except the boundary of time and the protected space that needs to be preserved from interruption, the aim of this group is not only to help interpersonal development but also to foster an awareness in both the individual and the group as a whole. This can lead to a sense of openness and shared responsibility for the functioning of the group. Exploration of individuals and their relationships to each other and to the group encourages an interest in new experiences.

Chris Rose (2008) writes:

> Working hard . . . is never enough on its own. Learning to understand and think about oneself requires a great deal more than an hour or so a week in term time only. It involves a commitment on the part of the students to take themselves very seriously indeed. This does not mean some dull earnestness, but rather a lively questioning of what we think we know about ourselves. We have ideas and pictures of who we are, what we are like, how we behave and how we relate that will all need revising . . . Taking oneself seriously means being alive to more possibilities than we had imagined and respecting our own capacity for creativity and flexibility.
>
> Rose (2008: 2–3)

Within this boundaried yet open environment of words and music, students can reflect on what it is like to train together in music therapy using the dual modality of words and music. It also gives them the opportunity to understand their reactions and responses to each other and the group-as-a-whole in a way that group members cannot do on their own: a chance to be open and alive to the dynamics, the thinking and the feeling of the group as well as the individual.

Unlike other more task-orientated groups, the experiential group has, at its core, the potential for its members to communicate in deeper, more personal and emotional ways with each other. In this sense, the group has similarities with a therapy group. In order to get the most out of the group, participants need to bring their 'whole' selves. This may be a risk, where some competitiveness between peers can be expected. But the more open students can be about themselves, the more they will personally get out of the group. This type of group offers the opportunity for individuals to grow in insight, as they negotiate their relationships with each other and the group-as-a-whole, seeing themselves from another person's point of view and recognising how they relate to others and others relate to them.

It would be natural for music therapists in training to ask at the beginning of training why there is a group like this. Questioning the purpose of the group is an important aspect of this type of group as well as an ongoing theme often revisited throughout the life of the group. Questions that may come up are: What is the purpose of the experiential group when there is no agenda except being in a designated place at and for a specific time? Why have a group of this kind on a training and why is it expected that all students should attend? As it is not assessed formally except in terms of attendance, why is the group considered to be one of the most important aspects of training in music therapy?

Students sometimes say that, if they are having their individual therapy whilst training, isn't that the place for learning about themselves? This, of course, is true. But we are not units in ourselves; we are part of a bigger society and whatever our own personal psychology, we all interact with others and have our being set firmly in the world with and in relation to other people. Foulkes, as we have seen earlier in the book, focused on the interconnectedness and the inter-relatedness of our experience and these dynamics are central to the exploration taking place in an experiential group.

I am often asked by students how their group compares with other groups I have facilitated. I sometimes respond by asking the group to reflect on why they ask the question. Do they fear that they may not live up to my, the conductor's, expectations? What are their thoughts, their fantasies? All I can say is that this combination of people, me included, are on a journey that has never been made before. In that sense, we are all on a level playing field. With this in mind, we will be in a unique situation together and it is up to every one of us to make of this something creative and meaningful. Students get the best out of the group if they are willing to be open to reflection and thoughtfulness about themselves and others as well as the group-as-a-whole. A certain curiosity is encouraged about how they and others participate in the group, both verbally and musically. This becomes fertile ground for self-development.

Groups can be very powerful places and the experiential group is no exception. They can engender feelings of love, acceptance and understanding. But they can also be places of strong feelings such as rivalry, envy, hate, contempt and misunderstanding. Witnessing empathic understanding as well as experiencing difficulties and how they may or may not be resolved can greatly enhance participants' personal growth as future music therapists and the work that they may do with groups themselves.

The individual and the group-as-a-whole

Sue Greenland (2002) draws attention to the way S.H. Foulkes locates the group at the centre of theory rather than the individual.

> Whilst acknowledging the clinical usefulness and relevance of the fundamental discoveries Freud brought to the individual psyche in terms of the unconscious processes, Foulkes invites us to look through a different lens and take the group as priority . . . although it is sometimes useful to separate the part from the whole, the individual from the group, in isolation they have no meaning.
>
> Greenland (2002: 275)

Foulkes (1948/1983) argues that:

> each individual – itself an artificial, though plausible, abstraction – is basically and centrally determined, inevitably, by the world in which he lives, by the community, the group, of which he forms part.
>
> Foulkes (1948/1983: 10)

How does this all apply to the experiential group and, in particular, one that uses music as well as talking as a currency of communication? The absence of a structure or a designated theme provokes anxiety and this in turn can bring out the true feelings and nature of people's relatedness and sense of themselves in the presence of others. Focussing on members' relatedness to each other helps towards thinking in terms of the group-as-a-whole. Relationships are very prominent in the improvised or more 'free associative' music in the group. It becomes clear who takes a leading role, either starting an improvisation or wanting to lead the group to new themes or dynamics. Observations in the music may reveal who might be more isolated, or who finds it difficult to relate to musical themes initiated by others. The music may also have the potential to bring the group together, as group members make an improvised piece that is the product of the whole group. Having experienced playing together, they can then reflect on the relationships that have taken place in the music.

Group improvisation can clarify the mood of the group that may be hard to get to in words. The music may also give the student, anxious about talking with others, a safer place for expression, and as George Steiner (1997) points out about music: 'Its forms in motion are at once more immediate and freer than those of language' (1997: 65).

An example

One student starts an improvisation on the drums using quite set rhythms and harmonic structures based of the sort of music she knows and could easily reproduce. The group acknowledges this and joins in with her. Another student, clearly irritated by this set, rather prescribed way of playing, introduces dissonance and cross rhythms in what appears to be a counter theme. What transpires is a lively Rondo (ABACADA) in which the conventional theme on the drums is returned to as something known whilst the interspersed musical episodes, mostly played on melodic instruments, represent the new and experimental diversions in the form of dissonance and alternative rhythms. The music was talked about afterwards in terms of the balance of the known with the unknown within the group and also on the training as a whole; what each member felt comfortable with and what they found more uncomfortable and challenging.

The matrix and the experiential group

Foulkes (1970/1990) discusses the network or web of relationships in the group which he called the 'matrix': 'an ever-expanding network of communication . . . the mother soil in which all dynamic processes take place' (1970/1990: 212).

Here is a reminder of how Foulkes described three forms of interlocking matrices. There is firstly the personal matrix, where the individual is formed and influenced by his early origins, in particular the family. Secondly there is the dynamic matrix which, in the context of the here-and-now of the group, is where each person's communication has both a personal and a group meaning. Third is the foundation matrix, which Foulkes describes as a broader matrix and is determined by both culture and biology.

These interlocking matrices can be seen to be at work within the experiential group. Each student, formed within their group of origin, their family, and from their unique musical experiences and heritage, brings a personal foundation matrix to the group. The dynamic matrix, informed by these matrices, is then re-constituted in the immediacy of the interactions that happen between each person as the group develops. Modification and new ways of relating may develop as members learn to relate communicatively through music, through language and by other non-verbal means such as gesture or attitude. Psyches formed within the matrix of family and within a person's own experience of music may be transformed and creatively adapted in the context of the group. New ways of relating can often take place when trainees struggle to find a way to be heard and understood by others and the group as a whole both in the music and in words.

It is also worth noting that, for some music therapy students, their early musical experiences have been fraught with anxiety relating to performance and other pressures. These can reveal themselves in the music but also ultimately be helped by the use of free improvisation where there is not necessarily a set idiom to adhere to. These are all part of the dynamic matrix that evolves in the group. Foulkes describes the dynamic matrix as 'ever-moving' and 'ever-developing' (1958/1990: 228).

Mirroring

Chris Rose (2008) writes: 'Just as we need some sort of reflection to see our physical selves and to build an internal image of how we look, we need reflections to develop the sense of our inner selves' (2008: 108).

Group members see in each other reflections of themselves, sometimes recognised and sometimes not. Foulkes (1948/1983) wrote: 'These neurotics are, after all, people like you and me and part of our annoyance is due to the fact that they show us our own weaknesses in a mirror – like a caricature' (1948/1983: 28).

We all have many facets to our personalities, and different groups, people and situations bring these out in each one of us. Rose (2008: 109) reminds us of the familiar example of the 'child' and the 'adult' self. Most adults can recognise a 'child' aspect to themselves that they find influences their behaviour at certain times. The experiential group can be a place where this 'inner child' in each one of us can be observed and where aspects of ourselves mingle and are brought out in relation to the many selves of others.

Sometimes a student in an experiential group may present one particular mode of being. They may be loud and dominating or over-anxious for something to happen. That could be reflected or mirrored in the music, perhaps in the form of not being able to leave space for others, and or becoming overwhelming with their musical contribution. Conversely, a student might present another or opposite side of themselves in the music or words. For instance a student, articulate and lively in words, may be more inhibited in the music, or a student very confident in the music may be less so in speaking. Having both modalities, that of words and music, gives a choice of expression and therefore alternative avenues through which to be understood.

Observations by all group members of these 'here-and-now' dynamics can help the individual and the group to a greater awareness. The conductor might initially point out some of these dynamics both in the speaking and in the music but the group members' growing ability to do the observing themselves has more of an impact in the group. It is no longer the authority figure of the conductor making the insights, but themselves as peers, increasingly becoming therapists for one another.

An example from the improvised music

A group member starts an improvisation and another member, echoing the same theme, joins in. The conductor notices that both these members are often validating or mirroring each other in the group. This dynamic is clearly being reproduced in the music. They play for quite a time, obviously enjoying the fact that they are playing in the same key and recognising the mutuality of dynamics and rhythm. Soon another member comes in with rhythmic music that is contrasting and introduces dissonance. The music continues with others joining in, in a way that both embraces the shared theme that was so noticeable with the first two players but also incorporates new and different musical ideas.

The discussion afterwards centres upon these elements of similarity and difference. Group members are able to link what happened in the music to the ideas of mirroring. They begin to exchange and discuss what they learnt about themselves and their reaction to others. Some see similar aspects of themselves in others that make them feel a sense of belonging and comfort. The idea of being challenged by differences is also something group members feel could enliven the group, just as the addition of dissonance seems to make the music much more interesting.

Resonance

Bill Lintott (2010 unpublished) writes:

> 'Resonance' describes the unique response of individual members to a shared group experience. Any group event, any subject discussed, will affect all, but not in the same way. Each member, reminded of past experience and influenced by assumptions formed earlier in life, will react in a way that is distinct from the others.
>
> Lintott (2010)

Resonance in a music therapy experiential group is nowhere better observed than in the music. Music played by one member is joined by, and has resonance with, another and is then perhaps developed and joined by others who take it off in various directions.

Another kind of resonance, however, is the unconscious connection between people. I am often aware, as a group conductor, of the sense that a member or members of the group can pick up what I am feeling and observing without my saying anything. The resonance is in the group matrix. What I am experiencing is most often others' experience too: an interconnectedness.

An example

A group was unusually silent. There was a real feeling of sadness present and this was clearly resonating between them at an unspoken level. I certainly felt it. I knew one of the members had experienced a bereavement, but no one was mentioning it. At my suggestion, the group began to improvise music together. The music was in a minor key; it was slow and expressive, using melodic instruments such as a metallophone and a lyre as well as the piano, and adding the eerie, gravelly sound of the ocean drum. This had a profound effect on the group. When the piece ended, the students thought together about what the music might have been expressing, all conscious of its poignancy. This created a sense of release and they were then able to speak about the sorrow that was there in the group but up until then had not been acknowledged. Group members expressed support for each other as they both acknowledged the particular member's loss but also shared their own experiences of bereavement. The music had resonated for them at a deep level. This group, initially frozen by a trauma that affected them all, melted into shared grief.

The music was the trigger to release the feeling that at some level they all shared. Words may have subsequently have been needed to state the grief and to name it but a shared, resonant, musical experience was really what connected them emotionally to each other.

Similarities and differences: inclusion and exclusion

Similarities and differences, and inclusion and exclusion are universal themes in groups and ones that are especially prominent in experiential group dynamics where students are training together. Observing similarities, difference, inclusion and exclusion, and the feelings that these evoke, can help towards more tolerance and understanding of others. Sharing and being able to listen to differences and consider other people's positions is invaluable learning. There is also the comfort at times of group members knowing that they are not alone in their experience and that others may have similar anxieties, hopes and fears.

The music can also have the potential to allow group members to feel that they are 'met' and supported. To be responded to or joined by others in the music can generate a feeling of acceptance. However, music can also be experienced as exclusive when, for instance, it might be difficult to have your contribution to the music heard because others are too loud, or certain subgroups of musicians play in a way that allows little opportunity for others to join in. Observing such dynamics and facilitating reflection and discussion about what is happening can bring a group to greater awareness of the dynamics that are present.

Potential confrontations and other difficult dynamics brewing in the group might also find safer expression in the music. Having had the feelings played in the music, some of these difficult issues can then be talked about or brought into thought more productively. In this way, playing music together can reveal dynamics in a less confrontational way.

An example

A student who had been quiet for most groups and who had not found it easy to join in the group conversation, suddenly came to life with her viola towards the end of the year, taking a prominent role in the improvised music. After playing what was a very expressive outpouring, she was then able to express in words her anxiety about speaking and about the exclusion she felt when others were so articulate. This led to others in the group acknowledging their own experience and fear of talking. It also helped those who found words easy to understand something of the difficulties of others.

For me, as conductor, witnessing this unfolding confirmed how music can provide an important means of getting to the feelings behind the words, allowing the communication to flow.

Transference and projection

Understanding transferences that reveal themselves in an experiential group can help members see where powerful emotions may be coming from. The most obvious areas of transference in a group are those rooted in the family of origin as well as other important figures, both benign and malignant, who have been part of a group member's upbringing. As Antony Powell (1994) points out:

> There is . . . in the analytic group a forum for a rich dramatisation of father, mother and sibling transferences, tending either towards the re-enactment of what once went before or, equally importantly, to a search for what was missing in the matrix of the family of origin.
>
> Powell (1994: 14)

Negative transferences in the experiential group situation, as opposed to individual therapy, can be easier to deal with. For one thing, there are more people present to think together about the transference phenomena. For the music therapy student, understanding transference can be a great asset in helping them to develop their clinical skills and sensitivities.

The question of how transference issues can get played out in the music is an interesting one. This may be useful to analyse, although sometimes leaving the music to speak for itself may be important. Juliet Alvin, one of the earliest pioneers in music therapy, is reported to have said that the instruments, and in particular the drum, could bear the brunt of a negative transference. This is an interesting observation, but it is also useful at times, having recognised what strong feelings may have been played out on the instruments, to describe them in words and see where their origin is. Words may aid thinking and thoughtfulness, but the music can recognise the feelings and be a channel for their expression.

The role of the conductor

The conductor in an experiential group is there primarily to hold the boundaries, especially those of time and space. This involves all that the conductor does to create and maintain the setting, such as dealing with absences, latecomers, communications outside the group, the institution, and the group timetable. What the conductor does in this respect, as dynamic administrator, is in the service of helping to stabilise the group, making it a safe container so that the dynamics or disturbances that emerge in the group can have the best possible chance of being understood and worked with.

The conductor of an experiential training group prepares the room for the students and seeks to keep the edges of the group safe from interruption. Preparation involves not only arranging seating but getting the instruments ready for use. Where possible, if students are able to leave the room as it is at the end of the session, they are also symbolically leaving aspects of the group dynamics in the room. They may then feel that they do not have to 'mop up' their feelings immediately, when they perhaps need time to process what has happened. Sometimes to be able to rush off or make a quick exit at the end of the group time is what a group member needs.

The conductor may observe how the instruments have been rearranged in a different way from the start of the session. For instance, the 'muddle' that the instruments have been left in might represent a disorder that was experienced in the group. Or maybe the instruments have been left untouched, which also might say something about that particular group. This is all useful for the conductor to observe after the session.

The role of the conductor is often the focus of the first few weeks in the group. 'Why aren't you doing anything?' 'Why aren't you telling us what to do?' are typical questions directed at the conductor, either explicitly or implicitly, as the anxiety of 'not knowing' builds up. If group members can be helped to hold this uncertainty, suspending judgement and preconceived ideas about the group, they may be able to let events unfold organically and thus be open to new experiences. Eventually, group members can learn to take ownership of the group and share the responsibility of enabling the group to function creatively.

An important role for the conductor in helping to maintain the boundaries that keep the group safe is to facilitate the group's consideration of and responsibility for matters such as confidentiality. As Lintott (2010) says:

> Consistency over time and place for sessions is the responsibility of the facilitator. Other boundaries are normally negotiated by the members in the course of discussion. Each will have an interest in maintaining confidentiality and they may share the wish that nothing said during sessions should be taken out of the group. They may expect that all communications will be shared and open to all, and so avoid meeting outside the sessions, while any who do meet will be expected to avoid discussing group matters. When boundaries are respected, confidence, trust and the 'containment' of the group will grow.
>
> Lintott (2010: 1)

It might be important to encourage the group to make their own rules, just as Lintott suggests, by negotiating with each other. Handing over this responsibility to the group for discussion becomes much more meaningful an experience for group members than attempting to dictate to them. Having some thoughts themselves around confidentiality and negotiating their own rules allows members to own the group. It also helps them to know what confidentiality both feels like and means for them rather than simply having an authority imposing rules from outside. On a music therapy training it is of course inevitable that members meet out of the group. However, the experience of holding confidentiality regarding group material becomes an important point of learning for therapy students as their future work will call for sensitivity to this issue. The task for the group is to learn how to manage this in the sometimes imperfect setting of a training.

An example of a boundary issue

The group had been going for about half an hour when an outsider burst into the room asking for music stands that he could see were in the back of the room. The conductor, rather taken aback, and not thinking, gestured to the intruder that he could help himself to the stands he wanted. The group was halted in its flow and when the person had left the room, group members looked to the conductor for an explanation. They were clearly affronted that the conductor had not protected the space. The conductor realising her mistake in not protecting the group against interruption apologised to the group and admitted to the group that she should have been more attentive. However, she was able to then explore the feeling of group members and their reaction to the incident. This proved a good learning situation. Some said they were shocked at the intrusion, but that the experience would help them as therapists to understand the importance of a protected space and what it might feel like if this space was not safe from interruption. Others were interested in the 'mistake' of the conductor in letting someone into the room whilst the group was going on and they felt cross. Some realised that even with experience, these lapses sometimes happen on the part of the conductor and if they were talked about and acknowledged, this could be an aspect of learning by experience for both the conductor and the group members.

Monitoring

For the conductor, maintaining free-floating attention or the ability to free associate can be a way of monitoring the pulse of the group: the complex, often seemingly chaotic conscious and unconscious communications expressed through words, music and other non-verbal means. The countertransference of the conductor is helpful to monitor too. When interweaving narratives are often very complex, countertransference sensitivity, combined with 'free-floating attention', offers the conductor useable data to help him/her understand what is going on in the group. Streeter (1995) used the term 'musical countertransference': 'The music therapist can examine her own responses to the role she takes within the music, what we call her musical countertransference, and in this way get a deeper sense of the client's inner experience' (1995: 40).

The same can be said for the conductor of a music therapy group. How she finds herself listening to or playing herself in a musical improvisation with the group can sensitise her to the mood, underlying atmosphere or hidden communications of the group.

Example 1

The conductor might pick up on a feeling that something important is not being said. She may perhaps experience some of the repressed or displaced anger that is coming from the group. There may be a complaint that one of the lecturers on the course is not keeping a good time boundary, is late for lectures and 'seemingly' not caring for them. At the same time one of the group members is always late whilst another often sends excuses that they have too much other course work on at the moment and need to be at home finishing their essay. The conductor, monitoring her own countertransference feelings of irritation and anger, has a strong feeling that the group is rather fed up with these group members and feels their lack of support and responsibility to the group but can't say so and finds it easier to transfer their anger onto the course tutors. The conductor monitors these projections and unspoken communication and holds them in mind. With any luck, the group members make this connection, maybe with some suggestion from the conductor. The focus is then on the here-and-now dynamic of the absent members which is then acknowledged as the source of the group's discontent, but which is harder to speak about.

Example 2

The group members are clearly angry about something but are not saying so. The conductor has a sense that there is a lot of anger expressed in the improvised music. She observes the clashes of harmony or the insistence on strong musical dynamics. She gets a sense that there is a holding back in the music and a musical explosion is about to erupt. She feels this by playing herself in the improvisation and attending to her musical countertransference: how she herself is feeling and responding in the music. She also senses an angry dynamic when she listens but does not play. She asks the group then to reflect on the music. They speak about how the music seems rather loud but do not make any link with the angry group dynamics the conductor senses. She monitors this as an aspect of the group that is not being talked about. At this point she intervenes with a suggestion that a sense of anger seems to have been around in the group from the beginning of the session. Gradually, with some reflection, group members agree that this was so and they then identify as the source of their feelings a particular incident on the course prior to the session, which had evoked very strong reactions.

Managing the transference

Although the transference towards the conductor does not, from a group analytic point of view, play as central a role as it does in individual therapy, it nevertheless has considerable significance and, within the context of the music therapy experiential group, offers opportunities for student learning. It is important, then, that the conductor allows time for the transference to emerge. However, the conductor is expected to hold, think about and feel the full impact of negative transferences towards her and this can be difficult.

By taking a stance of a relatively 'blank screen', where less is known about her, it is easier for this to happen and for fantasies to show themselves uninterrupted by reality checks and reason. When the transference towards the conductor is perceived by group members and subsequently worked with, group members are better able to understand not only aspects of their own relational patterns, in particular their ways of relating to authority, but also transferences in their own clinical practice. However, too much focus on the fantasies people have about the conductor may obscure other important issues that might be going on between group members. It is a question of balance.

A matter of balance

The art of the conductor lies in the balance between intervention and holding on and not outpacing the group. Insights that the group has come to from their own realisation are invariably more powerful than those from the conductor. Foulkes is well known to have advocated trusting the group rather than leading the group or treating the group in any way. The skill of the conductor rests in the ability to hold the balance between letting the group's own wisdom emerge and intervening in the service of helping the group find their own creative understanding of their process.

The maturing of the group

As the experiential group matures and develops, there is movement from the self or the individual as the reference point, towards the self in relation to the group. John Schlapobersky (1994) describes the progression in a group from speech patterns that are

> initially dominated by narrative and description to more mature forms that include reflective dialogue and discourse; and then a capacity to abstract and generalise from this experience, both inside and beyond the group. This progression recapitulates the child's primary pattern of growth in a decentring movement outward from the centre of the self ... The paradox of this progression is that, as the intersubjective domain is deepened and enriched, participants become more themselves by moving outward from themselves.
> Schlapobersky (1994: 215)

Endings

Endings have particular significance in a group that starts and finishes together. This has a parallel process with the ending of the training course itself. The conductor, alert to this importance, listens out for communications in the group material that consciously or unconsciously have to do with the ending of the group. For instance, one group might talk about their 'leaving home' experiences as teenagers or their particular anxiety about being out in the world of work without the support of the training course. It could then be productive to direct them to the 'here-and-now' of the group and explore their feelings about coming to the end of this group time with one other and what the loss of this space might mean.

This can be explored in the music where their experiences with each other, that might initially be hard to frame in words, can be expressed in the music. Group members' past experiences of endings, both good and bad, will often emerge, as will their sadness about parting from each other after the experiences they have shared. Thinking about each other's contribution, both musically and in words, can create a very intimate space at this time. What would they remember about each other? What aspects of the group were memorable and what might they take away with them and hold in mind? How does the present moment compare with their first meeting with each other? Have they changed their view or thoughts on the group and each other? What were the opportunities that they missed?

Conclusion

I return to the image of setting sail at the beginning of this chapter: the boat sailing out to sea, and the group in mid-ocean with the conductor as navigator together with the group members, steering the group towards their destination. If students have allowed themselves to be open to others and to the new experiences that the group had to offer during this journey, they will leave not only having learnt about themselves in relation to others, but having felt a sense of community, belonging and support. All of this will have complemented their theoretical learning on the course, preparing them for their own clinical work with groups in the future.

References

Abelin, E.L. (1971) 'The role of the father in the separation-individuation process', in J.B. McDevitt and C.F. Settlage (eds) *Separation-Individuation*, New York: International Universities Press.
— (1980) 'Triangulation, the role of the father and origin of core gender identity during the rapprochement sub-phase', in R.F. Lax, S. Bach, J.A. Burland (eds) *Rapprochement*, New York: Jason Aronson.
Agazarian, Y. and Gantt, S.P. (2000) *Autobiography of a Theory*, London: Jessica Kingsley Publishers.
Agazarian, Y. and Peters, R. (1981/1995) *The Visible and Invisible Group*, London: Karnac.
Ahonen-Eerikainen, H. (2011) *Group Analytic Music Therapy*, Philadelphia: Barcelona Publishers.
Aigen, K. (1996) *Being in Music – Foundations of Nordoff-Robbins Music Therapy*, St. Louis MO: MMB Music.
Anthony, E.J. (1983) 'The group-analytic circle and its ambient network', in M. Pines (ed.) *The Evolution of Group Analysis*, London: Routledge and Kegan Paul.
Argelander, H. (1970) 'Die szeishe Funktion des ich und ihr Anteil an der Symptom und Charakterbildung', *Psyche*, 24: 325–45.
Ashbach, C. and Schermer, V. (1987) *Object Relations, the Self, and the Group*, London: Routledge and Kegan Paul.
Bacal, H.A. (1985a) 'Object relations in the group from the perspective of self psychology', *International Journal of Group Psychotherapy*, 35: 483–501.
Bacal, H.A. (1985b) 'Optimal responsiveness and the therapeutic process', in A. Goldberg (ed.) *Progress in Self Psychology*, New York: Guildford Press.
— (1991) 'Reactiveness and responsiveness in the group therapeutic process', in S. Tuttman (ed.) *Psychoanalytic Group Theory and Therapy*, New York: International Universities Press.
— (1998) 'Notes on Optimal Responsiveness in the Group Process', in N.H. Harwood and M. Pines (eds) *Self Experiences in Group*, London: Jessica Kingsley Publishers.
Barenboim, D. (2001) 'Germans, Jews and Music', *New York Review of Books*, March 29th 2001.
Barnes, B., Ernst, S. and Hyde, K. (1999) *An Introduction to Groupwork*, London: Macmillan.
Baron-Cohen, S. (2003) *The Essential Difference*, New York: Basic Books,
Barwick, N. (2004) 'Bearing witness: group analysis as witness training in action', *Group Analysis*, 37: 121–36.

— (2006) 'Making room: developing reflective capacity through group analytic psychotherapy (part one)', *Psychodynamic Practice*, 12: 37–52.
Bateson, G. (1972) *An Ecology of Mind*, Chicago: University of Chicago Press.
— (1979) *Mind and Nature*, London: Wildwood House.
— (1994) 'Cohesive and disintegrative dynamics in group psychotherapy and their moderation by the leader', *Chinese Psychiatry*, 8: 69–82.
Battegay, R. (1994) 'Cohesive and disintegrative dynamics in group psychotherapy and their moderation by the leader', *Chinese Psychiatry*, 8: 69–82.
Beck, W. (2006) 'Countertransference in groups', *Group Analysis*, 39: 100–7.
Behr, H. (2004) 'Commentary on "Drawing the isolate into the group flow"', *Group Analysis*, 37: 76–81.
Behr, H. and Hearst, L. (2005) *Group-Analytic Psychotherapy*, London: Whurr.
Bennis, W.G. and Shephard, H.A. (1956) 'A theory of group development', *Human Relations*, 9: 415–37.
Bertalanffy, L. von (1968) *General Systems Theory*, revd edn, New York: George Braziller.
Bhaktin, M.M. (1986) *Speech Genres and Other Late Essays*, Austin, Texas: University of Texas Press.
Bion, W.R. (1959/1984) 'Attacks on linking', in *Second Thoughts*, London: Karnac.
— (1961) *Experiences in Groups*, London: Tavistock.
— (1962a/1984) 'A theory of thinking', in *Second Thoughts*, London: Karnac.
— (1970) *Attention and Interpretation*, London: Tavistock.
Blackwell, D. (1994) 'The psyche and the system', in D. Brown and L. Zinkin (eds) *The Psyche and the Social World*, London: Routledge.
Blunden, J. (2010) Cognitive Analytic Supervisory Training Days (unpublished)
Bollas, C. (1987) *The Shadow of the Object*, London: Free Association Books.
— (1989) *Forces of Destiny*, London: Free Association Books.
— (2000) *Hysteria*, London: Routledge.
— (2008) *The Evocative Object World*, Abingdon: Routledge.
Bowlby, J. (1973) *Attachment and Loss: Vol 2: Separation*, London: Hogarth Press
— (1979) *The Making and Breaking of Affectional Bonds*, London: Tavistock.
— (1988) *A Secure Base*, London: Routledge.
Britton, R. (1985/1992) 'The Oedipus situation and the depressive position', in R. Anderson (ed.) *Clinical Lectures on Klein and Bion*, London: Routledge.
— (1989) 'The missing link: parental sexuality in the Oedipus complex', in *The Oedipus Complex Today*, London: Karnac.
Brown, D. (1985/2000) 'Bion and Foulkes: basic assumptions and beyond' in M. Pines (ed.) *Bion and Group Psychotherapy*, London: Jessica Kingsley Publishers.
— (1986) 'Dialogue of change', *Group Analysis*, 19: 25–38.
— (1991) 'Assessment and selection for group', in J. Roberts and M. Pines (eds) *The Practice of Group Analysis*, London: Routledge.
— (2001) 'A contribution to the understanding of the social unconscious', *Group Analysis*, 34: 29–38.
— (2003) 'Pairing Bion and Foulkes' in R.M. Lipgar and M. Pines (eds) *Building on Bion: Roots*, London: Jessica Kingsley Publishers.
BSMT (1968) 'Pioneers in music therapy', *British Society of Music Therapy Bulletin*, 25: 18–19.
Burruth, M. (2008) 'Matriculating the matrix', *Group Analysis*, 41: 352–65.
Cage, J. (1968) *Silence*, London: Marion Boyars.

Cano, D.H. (1998) 'Oneness and Me-ness in the bag', in P. Bion Talamo, F. Borgogno and S.A. Merciai (eds) *Bion's Legacy to Groups*, London: Karnac.

Carr, C.E., d'Ardenne, P., Sloboda, A., Scott, C., Wang, D. and Priebe, S. (2012) 'Group music therapy for patients with persistent post-traumatic stress disorder – an exploratory randomized controlled trial with mixed methods evaluation', *Psychology and Psychotherapy: Theory, Research and Practice*, 85: 179–202.

Chazan, R. (2001) *The Group as Therapist*, London and Philadelphia: Jessica Kingsley Publishers.

Chused, J. and Raphling, C. (1992) 'The analyst's mistakes', *Journal of the American Psychoanalytic Association*, 40: 137–49.

Compton Dickinson, S.J. (2006) 'Beyond Body, Beyond Words: Cognitive analytic music therapy in forensic psychiatry- New approaches in the treatment of personality disordered offenders' Music Therapy Today Vol. V11 (4) 839–75. http://musictherapyworld.net (accessed 22/12/12).

Compton Dickinson, S.J., Adlam, J. and Odell-Miller, H. (2013) *Forensic Music Therapy: A treatment for men and women in secure hospital settings*, London: Jessica Kingsley Publishers.

Compton Dickinson, S.J. and Gahir, M. (2013) 'Working with Conflict: a summary of developments in the long-term treatment of a man suffering with paranoid schizophrenia who had committed manslaughter' in S.J. Compton Dickinson, J. Adlam, and H. Odell-Miller (eds) *Forensic music therapy: A treatment for men and women in secure hospital settings*, 121–137, London: Jessica Kingsley Publishers.

Cortesao, E.L. (1991) 'Group analysis and aesthetic equilibrium', *Group Analysis*, 24: 271–77.

Cozolino, L. (2006) *The Neuroscience of Human Relationships*, New York: Norton.

Dalal, F. (1998) *Taking the Group Seriously*, London: Jessica Kingsley Publishers.

—— (2001) 'The social unconscious: a post-Foulkesian perspective', *Group Analysis*, 34: 539–55.

—— (2002) *Race, Colour and the Process of Racialisation*, Hove: Brunner-Routledge.

Damasio, A. (1999) *The Feeling of What Happens*, New York: Harcourt.

Darnley-Smith, R. and Patey, H. (2003) *Music Therapy*, London: Sage.

Davies, A. and Richards, E. (1998) 'Music therapy in acute psychiatry: our experience of working as co-therapist with a group for patients from two neighbouring wards', *British Journal of Music Therapy*, 12(2): 53–59.

—— (2002) *Music Therapy and Group Work: Sound Company*, London: Jessica Kingsley Publishers.

De Maré, P.B. (1972) *Perspectives in Group Psychotherapy*, London: Allen and Unwin.

DeCasper, A.J. and Fifer, W.P. (1980). 'Of human bonding: newborns prefer their mothers' voices', *Science*, 208, 1174–6.

DeCasper, A.J. and Spence, M.J. (1986) 'Prenatal maternal speech influences newborns' perception', *Infant Behavior and Development*, 2: 133–50.

Deri, S. (1978) 'Transitional phenomena', in S.A. Grolnick, L. Barkin and W. Muensterberger (eds) *Between Reality and Fantasy*, New York: Jason Aronson.

Diel, P. (1980) *Symbolism in Greek Mythology*, Shambhala: Boufler and Hotton.

Donne, J. (24th January 1572–31 March 1631) London, England.

Duggan, C. et al. (2007) *A systematic review of the effectiveness of pharmacological and psychological treatments for those with personality disorders*, Nottinghamshire Healthcare NHS Trust / Institute of Mental Health.

Durkin, H.E. (1983) 'Some contributions of general systems theory to psychoanalytic group psychotherapy', in M. Pines (ed.) *The Evolution of Group Analysis*, London: Routledge and Kegan Paul.

Elias, N. (1969) 'Sociology and Psychiatry', in S.H. Foulkes and G.S. Prince (eds) *Psychiatry in a Changing Society*, London: Tavistock.

— (1989/1991) *The Symbol Theory*, London: Sage.

— (1939/2000) *The Civilizing Process*, trans. E. Jephcott, revd edn, Oxford: Blackwell.

Elias, N. and Scotson, J. (1965/1994) *The Established and the Outsiders*, London: Sage.

Eliot, T.S. (1922) *The Waste Land*, London: Faber.

Ettin, M.F. (1993) 'Links between group process and social, political, and cultural issues', in H.I. Kaplan and B.J. Sadock (eds) *Comprehensive Group Psychotherapy*, 3rd edn, Baltimore: Williams and Wilkins.

Ezriel, H. (1952) 'Notes on psychoanalytic group therapy', *Psychiatry*, 15: 119–26.

— (1973) 'Psychoanalytic group therapy', in L.R. Wolberg and E.K. Schwartz (eds) *Group Therapy*, New York: Stratton Intercontinental Medical.

Fonagy, P. *Attachment theory and psychoanalysis*, New York: 2011.

Fonagy, P., Gergely, G., Jurist, E. and Target, M. (2002) *Affect Regulation, Mentalization, and the Development of the Self*, New York: Other Press.

Foulkes, S.H. (1936/1990) 'Biology in the light of the work of Kurt Goldstein', in E. Foulkes (ed.) *Selected Papers*, London: Karnac.

— (1948) 'Introduction to group analytic therapy', in S. Mennell (1992) *Perspectives on Group Psychotherapy and Group Process*, London. Available online at onlinelibrary.wiley.com/doi/10.1002/9780470713006.biblio/pdf (accessed 14/06/2013).

— (1948/1983) *Introduction to Group-Analytic Psychotherapy*, London: Karnac.

— (1958/1990) 'Discussion of L.S. Kubie: some theoretical concepts underlying the relationship between individual and group psychotherapies', in E. Foulkes (ed.) *Selected Papers*, London: Karnac.

— (1964) *Therapeutic Group Analysis*, London: Allen and Unwin.

— (1968/1990) 'Group dynamic processes and group analysis', in E. Foulkes (ed.) *Selected Papers*, London: Karnac.

— (1970/1990) 'Access to unconscious processes in the group-analytic group', in E. Foulkes (ed.) *Selected Papers*, London: Karnac.

— (1971/1990) 'The group as matrix of the individual's mental life', in E. Foulkes (ed.) *Selected Papers*, London: Karnac.

— (1971/1990) 'Access to unconscious processes in the group-analytic group', in E. Foulkes (1974/1990) 'My philosophy in psychotherapy', in E. Foulkes (ed.) *Selected Papers*, London: Karnac.

— (1972/1990) 'Oedipus conflict and regression', in E. Foulkes (ed.) *Selected Papers*, London: Karnac.

— (1973/1990) 'The group as matrix of the individual's mental life', in E. Foulkes (ed.) *Selected Papers*, London: Karnac.

— (1975a/1986) *Group Analytic Psychotherapy*, London: Karnac.

— (1975b) 'A short outline of the therapeutic process in group-analytic psychotherapy', *Group Analysis*, 8: 59–63.

— (1977/1990) 'Notes on the concept of resonance', in E. Foulkes (ed.) *Selected Papers*, London: Karnac.

Foulkes, S.H. and Anthony, E.J. (1957) *Group psychotherapy: the psychoanalytic approach*, London: Karnac.

Foulkes, S.H. and Anthony, E.J. (1965/1984) *Group Psychotherapy*, 2nd ed. (rev. 1973), London: Karnac.
Freud, S. (1913/2002) 'On initiating treatment', trans. A. Bance, *Wild Analysis*, London: Penguin.
— (1915) 'The unconscious', S.E.14, 161–215.
— (1921/1991) 'Group psychology and the analysis of the ego', trans. A. Richards, *Sigmund Freud: 12*, Harmondsworth: Penguin.
— (1926) Letter to Trigant Burrow 14 November 1926, cited in J. Campos (1992), 'Burrow, Foulkes and Freud: An Historical Perspective', *Lifwynn Correspondence*, 2: 8.
Gans, J.S. (1989) 'Hostility in group psychotherapy', *International Journal of Group Psychotherapy*, 39: 499–516.
Gantt, S.P. and Hopper, E. (2008a) 'Two perspectives on a trauma in a training group: the systems-centred approach and the theory of incohesion: part I', *Group Analysis*, 41: 98–112.
— (2008b) 'Two perspectives on a trauma in a training group: the systems-centred approach and the theory of incohesion: part II', *Group Analysis*, 41: 123–39.
Garland, C. (1982) 'Group-analysis: taking the non-problem seriously', *Group Analysis*, 15: 4–14.
George, C., Kaplan, N. and Main, M. (1985) *The Berkely Adult Attachment Interview*, University of California. Available online at http://www.psychology.sunysb.edu/attachment/measures/content/aai_interview.pdf (accessed 20/02/2013).
Gergely, G. et al (1995) 'Taking the intentional stance at 12 months of age', *Cognition*, 56: 165–93.
Gergely, G. and Watson, J.S. (1999). 'Early social-emotional development: contingency, perception and social feedback model', in P. Rochat (ed.) *Early Social Cognition*, 101–36. Hillside, NJ.
Gerson, S. (2004) 'The relational unconscious', *Psychoanalytic Quarterly*, 73: 63–98.
Gibbard, G.S. and Hartman, J.J. (1973) 'The significance of utopian fantasies in small groups', *International Journal of Group Psychotherapy*, 23: 125–47.
Good Reads: http://www.goodreads.com/author/quotes/54761.Miles_Davis (accessed 02/04/2013).
Gordon, J. (1994) 'Bion's post-*Experiences in Groups* thinking on groups', in V.L. Schermer and M. Pines (eds) *Ring of Fire*, London: Routledge.
Green, L. (1983) 'On fusion and individuation processes in small groups', *International Journal of Group Psychotherapy*, 33: 3–19.
Greenland, S. (2002) 'A group analytic look at experiential groups', in A. Davies and E. Richards *Music Therapy and Group Work: Sound Company*, London: Jessica Kingsley Publishers.
Grotjahn, M. (1977) *The Art and Technique of Analytic Group Therapy*, New York: Jason Aronson.
Grotstein, J.S. (1981) 'Wilfred Bion: the man, the psychoanalyst, the mystic' in J.S. Grotstein (ed.) *Do I Dare Disturb the Universe?*, Beverley Hill: Caesura Press.
Guntrip, H. (1975) 'My experience of analysis with Fairbairn and Winnicott', *International Review of Psycho-Analysis*, 2: 145–56.
Hall, T.W. (2007) 'Psychoanalysis, attachment and spirituality', *Journal of Psychology and Theology*, 35: 14–28.
Harris, T. (1992) 'Some reflections on the process of social support and the nature of unsupportive behaviour', in H.O.F. Veiel and E. Baumann (eds) *The meaning and measurement of social support*, Washington: Hemisphere Publishing Corporation.

Harwood, I. (1986) 'The need for optimal, available selfobject caretakers', *Group Analysis*: 19: 291–302.

Heal, M. (1989) 'In tune with the mind', in D. Brandon (ed.) *Mutual Respect: therapeutic approaches to working with people who have learning difficulties*, Surbiton: Good Impressions.

— (1992) 'A comparison of mother-infant interactions and the client-therapist relationship in music therapy sessions', in T. Wigram, R. West, and B. Saperston, (eds) *Music and the Healing Processes*, London: Carden.

Hinshelwood, R. (1994) 'Attacks on the reflective space', in V.L. Schermer and M. Pines (eds) *Ring of Fire*, London: Routledge.

— (2007) 'Bion and Foulkes', *Group Analysis*, 40: 344–56.

Hobson, R.P. and Kapur, R. (2005) 'Working in the transference', *Psychology and Psychotherapy*, 78: 275–93.

Holmes, J. (1996) *Attachment, intimacy, autonomy*, New Jersey: Jason Aronson.

— (2001) *The Search for the Secure Base*, London: Routledge.

— (2002) 'Are poetry and psychotherapy too "wet" for serious psychiatrists?' *The Psychiatrist*, 26: 138–40.

Hopper, E. (1997) 'Traumatic experience in the unconscious life of groups: a fourth basic assumption', *Group Analysis*, 30: 439–70.

— (2001) 'The social unconscious', *Group Analysis*, 34: 9–27.

— (2002) 'Letter to the editor commenting on: "The social unconscious: a post-Foulkesian perspective" (by Farhad Dalal)', *Group Analysis*, 35: 333–35.

— (2003a) *The Social Unconscious*, London: Jessica Kingsley.

— (2003b) *Traumatic Experience in the Unconscious Life of Groups*, London: Jessica Kingsley.

— (2006) 'Theoretical and conceptual notes concerning transference and countertransference processes in groups and by groups, and the social unconscious, part I', *Group Analysis*, 39: 549–59.

— (2007) 'Theoretical and conceptual notes concerning transference and countertransference processes in groups and by groups, and the social unconscious, part II', *Group Analysis*, 40: 21–34.

— (2009) 'The theory of the basic assumption of incohesion: aggregation/massification or (Ba) I:A/M, *British Journal of Psychotherapy*, 25: 214–29.

Hopper, E. and Weinberg, H. (2011) *The Social Unconscious in Persons, Groups and Societies: vol. 1*, London: Karnac.

Horwitz, L. (1977) 'A group-centered approach to group psychotherapy', *International Journal of Group Psychotherapy*, 27: 423–39.

Hudson, I. (2008) 'Do group analysts have to go it alone? In praise of co-therapy'. Unpublished paper.

Hutchinson, S. (2009) 'Foulkesian authority', *Group Analysis*, 42: 354–60.

Jacobson, L. (1989) 'The group as an object in the cultural field', *International Journal of Group Psychotherapy*, 39: 475–98.

James, C.D. (1982) 'Transitional phenomena and the matrix in group psychotherapy', in M. Pines and L. Rafalson (eds) *The Individual and the Group*, London: Plenum Press.

— (1984) 'Bion's "containing" and Winnicott's "holding" in the context of the group matrix', *International Journal of Group Psychotherapy*, 34: 1–13.

— (1994) '"Holding" and "Containing" in the group and society', in D. Brown and L. Zinkin (eds) *The Psyche and the Social World*, London: Routledge.

John, D. (1992) 'Towards music psychotherapy', *The Journal of British Music Therapy*, 6: 12.
Joseph, B. (1985) 'Transference – the total situation', *International Journal of Psycho-Analysis*, 66: 447–54.
Jung, C. (1968/1991) *Archetypes and the Collective Unconscious*, 2nd edition, trans. R.F.C. Hull, London: Routledge.
Karterud, S. (2011) 'Constructing and mentalizing the matrix', *Group Analysis*, 44: 357–73.
Kennard, D., Roberts, J. and Winter, D. (1990) 'What do group-analysts say in their groups?', *Group Analysis*, 23: 173–90.
—— (1993) *A Workbook of Group Analytic Interventions*, London: Routledge.
Kernberg, O. (1965) 'Notes on countertransference', *Journal of the American Psychoanalytic Association*, 13: 38–56.
Klein, M. (1929/1988) 'Infantile anxiety-situations reflected in a work of art and in the creative impulse', in *Love, Guilt and Reparation*, London: Virago Press.
—— (1946/1988) 'Notes on some schizoid mechanisms', in *Envy and Gratitude*, London: Virago Press.
—— (1952/1988) 'Some theoretical conclusions regarding the emotional life of the infant', in *Envy and Gratitude*, London: Virago Press.
Knoblauch, S. (2000) *The musical edge of therapeutic dialogue*, London: Routledge.
Kohut, H. (1971) *The Analysis of the Self*, New York: International Universities Press.
—— (1977) *The Restoration of the Self*, New York: International Universities Press.
—— (1984) *How Does Analysis Cure?* Chicago: University of Chicago Press.
Kosseff, J.W. (1975) 'The leader using object-relations theory', in Z.A. Liff and J. Aronson (eds) *The Leader in the Group*, New York: Jason Aronson.
Lavie, J. (2005) 'The lost roots of the theory of group analysis: "Taking interrelational individuals seriously"!', *Group Analysis*, 38: 519–35.
—— (2007) '"Open People", "Homo Clausus" and the "5th Basic Assumption": Bridging concepts between Foulkes's and Bion's traditions', *Funzione Gamma*. Available online at: http://www.funzionegamma.it/wp-content/uploads/open-people-19e.pdf (accessed 03/12/2012).
Lawrence, W.G., Bain, A. and Gould, L. (1996/2000) 'The fifth basic assumption', in W.G. Lawrence *Tongued with Fire*, London and New York: Karnac.
—— (2003) 'Narcissism v. Social-ism Governing Thinking in Social Systems', in R.M.
Levine, C.O. and Dang, J.C. (1979) 'The group within the group', *International Journal of Group Psychotherapy*, 29: 175–84.
Levine, S. (1997) *Poiesis: the language of psychology and the speech of the soul*, London: Jessica Kingsley Publishers.
Lewin, K. (1951) *Field Theory in Social Science*, New York: Harper and Row.
Lintott, W. (2010) *Group Analysis and Experiential Groupwork: A Cambridge Perspective*. Resource book for Madingly Counselling Course. Cambridge (unpublished).
Lipgar and M. Pines (eds) *Building on Bion: Branches*, London: Jessica Kingsley Publishers.
Maar, V. (1989) 'Attempts at grasping the self during the termination phase of group-analytic psychotherapy', *Group Analysis*, 22: 99–104.
Malan, D. (1979) *Individual Psychotherapy and the Science of Psychodynamics*, London: Butterworth.
Malan, D.H., Balfour, F.G.H., Hood, V.G., and Shooter, A.M.N. (1976) 'Group psychotherapy: a long-term follow-up study', *Archives of General Psychiatry*, 33: 1303–15.

Malinowski, B. (1923) 'The problem of meaning in primitive languages', in C.K. Ogden and I.A. Richards (eds), *The Meaning of Meaning: a study of the influence of language upon thought*, London: Routledge and Kegan Paul.

Markova, G. and Legerstee, G. (2006). 'Contingency, imitation and affect sharing: foundations of infants' social awareness', *Developmental Psychology*, 42, 132–41.

Marrone, M. (1994) 'Attachment theory and group analysis', in D. Brown and L. Zinkin (eds) *The Psyche and the Social World*, London: Routledge.

— (1998) *Attachment and Interaction*, London: Jessica Kingsley.

Marsh, L.C. (1933) 'An experiment in group treatment of patients at Worcester State Hospital', *Mental Hygiene*, 17: 396–416.

Mcgee, T. and Schuman, B.J. (1970) 'The nature of the co-therapy relationship', *The International Journal of Group Psychotherapy*, 20: 25–36.

Mead, G.H. (1934) *Mind, Self and Society*, C. W. Morris (ed.) Chicago: Chicago University Press.

Meltzer, D. (1968) *The Psycho-Analytic Process*, Perth: Clunie.

Meltzoff, A.N. and Gopnik, A. (1993). 'The role of imitation in understanding persons and developing theories of mind', in S. Baren-Cohen, H. Tager Fusberand and D. Cohen (eds) *Understanding Other Minds: perspectives from autism*, 335–66. Oxford: Oxford University Press.

Mendez, C.L., Coddou, F. and Maturana, H. (1988) 'The bringing forth of pathology', *Irish Journal of Psychology*, 9.

Merleau-Ponty, M. (1964) *The Primacy of Perception*, Evanston: Northwestern University Press.

Miller, J.G. (1969) 'Living systems: basic concepts', in W. Gray, L. Duhl, and N. Rizzo (eds) *General Systems Theory and Psychiatry*, Boston: Little Brown.

Morgan, G. (1986) *Images of Organization*, Beverley Hills, CA and London: Sage.

Nava, A.S. (2007) 'Empathy and group analysis', *Group Analysis*, 40: 13–28.

Neumann, E. (1963) *The Great Mother*, London: Routledge and Kegan Paul.

Nicolis, G. and Prigogine, I. (1989) *Exploring Complexity*, New York: W.H. Freeman and Co.

Nitsun, M. (1989) 'Early development: linking the individual and the group', *Group Analysis*, 22: 249–60.

— (1991) 'The anti-group: destructive forces in the group and their therapeutic potential', *Group Analysis,* 24: 7–20.

— (1994) 'The primal scene in group analysis', in D. Brown and L. Zinkin (eds) *The Psyche and the Social World*, London: Routledge.

— (1996) *The Anti-Group*, London: Routledge.

— (2009) 'Authority and revolt: the challenges of group leadership', *Group Analysis*, 42: 325–48.

Nordoff, P. and Robbins, C. (1973) *Therapy in Music for the Handicapped Child*, London: Victor Gollancz.

Odell-Miller, H. (2001) 'Music therapy and its relationship to psychoanalysis', in Y. Searle and I. Streng (eds) *Where Analysis Meets The Arts*, London: Karnac.

— (2013) 'Inside and outside the walls: music therapy supervision in a forensic setting', in S.J. Compton Dickinson, J. Adlam and H. Odell-Miller (eds) *Forensic Music Therapy: A treatment for men and women in secure hospital settings*, 43–58, London: Jessica Kingsley Publishers.

Ogden, T.H. (1979) 'On projective identification', *International Journal of Psycho-Analysis*, 60: 357–73.

— (1992a) 'The dialectically constituted/decentred subject of psychoanalysis, I', *International Journal of Psycho-Analysis*, 73: 517–26.
— (1992b) 'The dialectically constituted/decentred subject of psychoanalysis, II', *International Journal of Psycho-Analysis*, 73: 613–26.
— (2004) 'The analytic third', *Psychoanalytical Quarterly*, 73: 167–95.
Orange, D.M. (2009) 'The face of the other: beyond individuality in psychotherapy and psychoanalysis', presented at the *International Association of Psychoanalytic Self Psychology Annual Conference*, Chicago.
Ormont, L.R. (2004) 'Drawing the isolate into the group flow', *Group Analysis*, 37: 65–76.
Ornstein, P. (1981) 'The bipolar self in the psychoanalytic treatment process', *Journal of the American Psychoanalytic Association*, 2: 353–75.
Padel, J. (1985) 'Ego in current thinking', *International Review of Psychoanalysis*, 12: 273–83.
Pavlicevic, M. (1997) *Music Therapy in Context*, London: Jessica Kingsley Publishers.
— (2003) *Groups in Music: strategies from music therapy*, London: Jessica Kingsley Publishers.
Pines, M. (1978) 'Group analytic psychotherapy of the borderline patient', *Group Analysis*, 11: 115–26.
— (1982/1998) 'Reflections on mirroring', in *Circular Reflections*, London: Jessica Kingsley Publishers.
— (1983) 'On mirroring in group psychotherapy', *Group*, 7: 3–17.
— (1984/1998) 'Group analytic psychotherapy and the borderline patient', in *Circular Reflections*, London: Jessica Kingsley.
— (1985a/1998) 'Psychic development and the group analytic situation', in *Circular Reflections*, London: Jessica Kingsley Publishers.
— (1985b/1998) 'Mirroring and child development', in *Circular Reflections*, London: Jessica Kingsley Publishers.
— (1993) 'Interpretation: Why, for whom and when', in D. Kennard, J. Roberts and D. A. Winter, *A Work Book of Group-Analytic Interventions*, London: Routledge.
— (2003a) 'Social brain and social group: how mirroring connects people', *Group Analysis*, 36: 507–13.
— (2003b) 'Bion and Foulkes on empathy' in R.M. Lipgar and M. Pines (eds) *Building on Bion: Roots*, London and New York: Jessica Kngsley.
Pines, M., Hearst, L. and Behr, H. (1982) 'Group Analysis', in G.M. Garza (ed.) *Basic Approaches to Group Psychotherapy and Counseling*, 3rd edn, Springfield, IL: Charles Thomas.
Pinson, J. (2013) *Involving Senior Citizens In Group Music Therapy*, London: Jessica Kingsley Publishers.
Powell, A. (1983) 'The music of the group: a musical enquiry into group-analytic psychotherapy', *Group Analysis*, 16: 3–19.
— (1991) 'Matrix, mind and matter', *Group Analysis*, 24: 299–322.
— (1994) 'Towards a unifying concept of the group matrix', in D. Brown and L. Zinkin (eds) *The Psyche and the Social World*, London: Routledge.
Preston, S.D. and de Waal, F.B.M. (2002) 'Empathy: its ultimate and proximate bases', *Behavioural and Brain Sciences*, 25: 1–72.
Priestley, M. (1975) *Music Therapy in Action*, London: Constable.
— (1994) *Analytical Music Therapy*, Philadelphia: Barcelona Publishers.
— (1996) 'Linking sound and symbol', in T. Wigram, B. Saperston, R. West *The Art and Science of Music Therapy: A Handbook*, London: Routledge.

Prinz, W. (1997) 'Perception and action planning', in *European Journal of Cognitive Psychology*, 9: 129–54.

Prodgers, A. (1990) 'The dual nature of the group as mother: the uroboric container', *Group Analysis*, 23: 17–23.

—— (1991) 'Countertransference: The conductor's emotional response within the group setting', *Group Analysis*, 24: 389–407.

Qinodoz, D. (2009) *Growing Old: A journey of self-discovery*, London: Routledge.

Quintaneiro, T. (2004) 'The concept of figuration or configuration in Norbert Elias's sociological theory', trans. M. Mitre (2006) *Teoria and Sociedade*, Belo Horizonte, 12: 54–69. Available online at: http://socialsciences.scielo.org/scielo.php?pid=s1518-44712006000200002andscript=sci_arttext (accessed 05/11/2012).

Ramey, M. (2011) *Group Music Activities for Adults with Intellectual and Developmental Disabilities*, London: Jessica Kingsley Publishers.

Raphael-Leff, J. (1984) 'Myths and modes of motherhood', *British Journal of Psychotherapy*, 1: 14–18.

Rippa, B. (1994) 'Groups in Israel during the Gulf War', *Group Analysis*, 27: 87–94.

Rizzolatti, G., Fogassi, L. and Gallese, V. (2001) 'Neurophysiological mechanisms underlying the understanding and imitation of action', *Nature Review Neuroscience*, 2: 661–70.

Roberts, J. (1983) 'Foulkes's concept of the matrix', *Group Analysis*, 15: 111–26.

—— (1991) 'Destructive phases in groups', in J. Roberts and M. Pines (eds) *The Practice of Group Analysis*, London: Routledge.

Roberts, J. and Pines, M. (1992) 'Group-analytic psychotherapy', *International Journal of Group Psychotherapy*, 42: 469–94.

Roberts, R. (2013) 'Music, mourning and the matrix: death and loss within a forensic music therapy group', in S.J. Compton Dickinson, J. Adlam and H. Odell-Miller (eds) *Forensic Music Therapy: A treatment for men and women in secure hospital settings*, 137–54, London: Jessica Kingsley Publishers.

Rogers, C. (1987) 'On putting it into words: the balance between projective identification and dialogue in the group', *Group Analysis*, 20: 99–107.

Rose, C. (2008) *The Personal Development Group*, London: Karnac.

Rosenthal, L. (1987) *Resolving Resistances in Group Psychotherapy*, New Jersey: Jason Aronson.

Rycroft, C. (1985) *Psycho-analysis and Beyond*, London: Hogarth Press.

Ryle, A. and Kerr, I. (2002) *Introducing Cognitive Analytic Therapy*, Chichester: Wiley.

Sandler, J., Dare, C. and Holder, A. (1973) *The Patient and the Analyst*, London: Allen and Unwin.

Scheidlinger, S. (1964) 'Identification, the sense of belonging and of identity, in small groups', *International Journal of Group Psychotherapy*, 14: 291–306.

Schermer, V.L. (1985/2000) 'Beyond Bion: the basic assumption states revisited', in M. Pines (ed.) *Bion and Group Psychotherapy*, London: Jessica Kingsley Publishers.

—— (2010a) 'Reflections on "Reflections on mirroring"', *Group Analysis*, 43: 214–27.

—— (2010b) 'Mirror neurons: their relevance for group psychotherapy', *International Journal of Group Psychotherapy*, 60: 485–511.

—— (2012a) 'Group-as-a-whole and complexity theories: part I', *Group Analysis*, 45: 275–88.

— (2012b) 'Group-as-a-whole and complexity theories: part II', *Group Analysis*, 45: 481–97.
Schlachet, P. (1986) 'The concept of group space', *International Journal of Group Psychotherapy*, 36: 33–53.
Schlapobersky, J. (1994) 'The language of the group: monologue, dialogue and discourse in group analysis', in D. Brown and L. Zinkin (eds) *The Psyche and the Social World*, London: Routledge.
Schlapobersky, J. and Pines, M. (2009) 'Group methods in adult psychiatry' in M. Gelder, N. Andreasen, J. Lopez-Ibor and J. Geddes (eds) *The New Oxford Textbook of Psychiatry*, Oxford: Oxford University Press.
Scholz, R. (2003) 'The foundation matrix', *Group Analysis*, 36: 48–54.
Se Cho, Wook (2013) 'Gentling the bull: harnessing anti-group forces in music therapy group work with adults with learning disabilities', *BJMT*, 27: 6–15.
Segal, H. (1977) 'Countertransference', *International Journal of Psychoanalytic Psychotherapy*, 6: 31–7.
Segalla, R. (2012) 'The therapeutic work of the group: finding the self through finding the other', in I. Harwood, W. Stone and M. Pines (eds) *Self Experiences in Group, Revisited*, New York and London: Routledge.
Slavendy, J.T. (1993) 'Selection and preparation of patients and organisation of the group', in H.J. Kaplan and B.J. Sadock (eds) *Comprehensive Group Psychotherapy*, 3rd edn, Baltimore: Williams and Wilkins.
Sleight, V. and Compton Dickinson, S.J. (2013) 'Risks, ruptures and the role of the co-therapist: Group Cognitive Analytic Therapy (G-CAMT) a pilot group at a high secure hospital', in S.J. Compton Dickinson, J. Adlam and H. Odell-Miller (eds) *Forensic Music Therapy: A treatment for men and women in secure hospital settings*, 169–184, London: Jessica Kingsley Publishers.
Smith, K.K. and Berg, D.N. (1988) *Paradoxes of Group Life*, London: Jossey-Bass.
Spiegelman, J.M. and Mansfield, V. (1996) 'On the physics and psychology of the transference as an interactive field', *Journal of Analytical Psychology*, 41: 179–202.
Stacey, R. (2000) 'Reflexivity, self-organization and emergence in the group matrix', *Group Analysis*, 33: 501–14.
— (2001) 'Complexity theory and the group matrix', *Group Analysis*, 34: 221–40.
— (2003) *Complexity and Group Processes*, London: Brunner-Routledge.
— (2005) 'Affects and cognition in a social theory of unconscious processes', *Group Analysis*, 38: 159–76.
Stein, A. (1999) 'Well tempered bagatelles: a meditation on listening in psychoanalysis and music', *American Imago*, 56 (4): 397–416.
Stein, M. (ed.) (1995) *The Interactive Field in Analysis*, Wilmette, IL: Chiron.
Steiner, G. (1998) *Errata: An examined life*, Phoenix: London.
Stern, D. (1985) *The Interpersonal World of the Infant*, New York: Basic Books.
— (2004) *The Present Moment in Psychotherapy and Everyday Life*, New York: Norton.
— (2010) *Forms of Vitality*, Oxford: Oxford University Press.
Stern, D., Sandler, L.W., Nahum, J.P., Harrison, A.M., Lyons-Ruth, K. Morgan, A.C., Bruschweiler-Stern, N. and Tronick, E.Z. (1998) 'Non-interpretative mechanisms in psychoanalytic therapy', *International Journal of Psycho-Analysis*, 79: 903–21.
Stolorow, R.D., Brandchaft, B. and Atwood, G E. (1987) *Psychoanalytic Treatment: an intersubjective approach*, Hillsdale, NJ: Analytic Press.

Stone, E. (2001) 'Culture, politics and group therapy', *Group Analysis*, 34: 501–14.
Storr, A. (1992) *Music and the mind*, New York: Ballantine.
Streeter, E. (1987) 'Foreword', *Journal of British Music Therapy*, 1 (2): 3.
— (1995) 'Talking and playing: The dynamic relationship', *Journal of the Institute of Psychotherapy and Counselling*, 3: 4.
Strich, S. (1983) 'Music and the patterns of human interactions', *Group Analysis*, 16, 20–29.
Symington, N. (1986) *The Analytic Experience*, London: Free Association Books.
Thornton, C. (2004) 'Borrowing my self: an exploration of exchange as a group-specific therapeutic factor', *Group Analysis*, 37: 305–20.
Thygesen, B. (2008) 'Resonance: no music without resonance – without resonance no group', *Group Analysis*, 41: 63–83.
Towse, E. (1991) 'Relationships in music therapy: do music therapy techniques discourage the emergence of transference?' *British Journal of Psychotherapy*, 7 (4): 323–33.
Trevarthen, C. (1977) 'Descriptive analyses of infant communicative behaviour', in H.R. Schaffer (ed.) *Studies in Mother-Infant Interaction*, New York: Academic Press.
Tubert-Oklander, J. (2010) 'The matrix of despair: from despair to desire through dialogue', *Group Analysis*, 43: 127–40.
Tuckman, B. (1965) 'Developmental sequences in small groups', *Psychological Bulletin*, 63: 384–99.
Turquet, P. (1974) 'Leadership: the individual and the group', in G.S. Gibbard, J.J. Hartman and R.D. Mann (eds) *Analysis of the Group*, San Francisco: Jossey-Bass.
Tuttman, S. (1994) 'Therapeutic responses to the expression of aggression by members in groups', in V.L. Schermer and M. Pines (eds) *Ring of Fire*, London: Routledge.
Vella, N. (1999) 'Freud on groups', in C. Oakley (ed.) *What is a Group?*, London: Rebus Press.
Volkan, V.D. (2001) 'Transgenerational transmissions and chosen traumas: an aspect of large group identity', *Group Analysis*, 34: 79–97.
Vygotsky, L.S. (1962) *Thought and Language*, Cambridge, MA: MIT Press.
Wallin, D. (2007) *Attachment in Psychotherapy*, New York and London: Guilford Press.
Walrond-Skinner, S. (1976) *Family Therapy: The treatment of natural systems*. London. Routledge and Kegan Paul.
Ward, D. (1989) 'The termination process in the group process', *Group Analysis*, 22: 87–99.
Weinberg, H. (2007) 'So what is the social unconscious anyway?', *Group Analysis*, 40: 307–22.
Weinberg, H. and Toder, M. (2004) 'The hall of mirrors in small, large and virtual groups', *Group Analysis*, 37: 492–507.
Whitaker, D.S. and Lieberman, M.A. (1964) *Psychotherapy through the Group Process*, New York: Prentice-Hall.
Winnicott, D.W. (1947/1992) 'Hate in the countertransference', in *Through Paediatrics to Psycho-Analysis*, London: Karnac.
— (1951/1992) 'Transitional objects and transitional phenomena', in *Through Paediatrics to Psycho-Analysis,* London: Karnac.
— (1954/1992) 'Metapsychological and clinical aspects of regression within the psychoanalytical set-up' in *Through Paediatrics to Psycho-Analysis*, London: Karnac.

— (1956/1992) 'Primary maternal preoccupation' in *Through Paediatrics to Psycho-Analysis*, London: Karnac.
— (1960/1990) 'The theory of the parent-infant relationship', in *The Maturational Processes and the Facilitating Environment*, London: Karnac.
— (1964) *The Child, the Family and the Outside World*, London: Karnac.
— (1963/1990) 'Development of the capacity for concern', in C. Winnicott, R. Shepherd and M. Davis (eds) *Deprivation and Delinquency*, London: Routledge.
— (1964/1991) 'Roots of aggression', in *The Child, The Family, and the Outside World*, Harmondsworth: Penguin.
— (1965/1989) 'The relationship of a mother to her baby at the beginning', in *The Family and Individual Development*, London: Routledge.
— (1968/1989) 'The Squiggle Game', in C. Winnicott, R. Shepherd and M. Davis (eds) *Psycho-Analytic Explorations*, London: Karnac.
— (1971/1974) *Playing and Reality*, Harmondsworth: Pelican.
Wolf, E.S. (1980) 'On the developmental line of selfobject relations', in A. Goldberg (ed.) *Advances in Self Psychology*, New York: International Universities Press.
— (1988) *Treating the Self*, New York: Guildford Press.
Woodcock, J. (1987) 'Towards group analytic music therapy', *Journal of British Music Therapy*, 1: 16–21.
Wooster, G. (1983) 'Resistance in groups as developmental difficulty in triangulation', *Group Analysis*, 16: 30–40.
Wright, K. (1998) 'Deep calling unto deep: Artistic creativity and the maternal object', *British Journal of Psychotherapy*, 4: 453–67.
— (2009) *Mirroring and Attunement*, London: Routledge.
Yalom, I.D. (1985) *The Theory and Practice of Group Psychotherapy*, 3rd edn, Basic Books.
Yogev, H. (2008) 'Holding in relational theory and group analysis', *Group Analysis*, 41: 373–90.
— (2012) 'The capacity to be with', *Group Analysis*, 45: 339–57.
— (2013) 'The development of empathy and group analysis', *Group Analysis*, 46: 61–80.
Zinkin, L. (1983) 'Malignant mirroring', *Group Analysis*, 16: 113–26.
— (1989) 'The group as container and contained', *Group Analysis*, 22: 227–34.
— (1991) 'The Klein Connection in the London School: The Search for Origins', *Journal of Analytical Psychology*, 36: 37–61.
— (1994) 'Exchange as a therapeutic factor in group analysis', in D. Brown and L. Zinkin (eds) *The Psyche and the Social World*, London: Routledge.
— (1998) *Dialogue in the Analytic Setting*, London: Jessica Kingsley Publishers.

Index

Note: 'n' after a page number indicates a note.

Adorno, Theodor 48
adversarial needs 73
affect attunement: definition of 95; and mother–infant relationship 95–7, 117; and music therapy 97; and vitality affects 96. *See also* attunement
affect-sharing 74
Agazarian, Y. 86
aggregation/massification 82–3, 88n2
aggression: and anti-groups 85; and incohesion and aggregation 83
Ainsworth, Mary 104
Al-Farabi x
Alvin, Juliet 4, 12, 13, 14, 157
amplification and condenser phenomenon 40
AMT. *See* Analytical Music Therapy (AMT)
Analytical Music Therapy (AMT) 4, 5–6. *See also* Priestley, Mary
Anglia Ruskin University 12
Anthony, E. J.: on amplification and condenser phenomenon 40; on anti-group 85; on group communication 40; on mirroring 42; on resonance 38–9
anti-group: in case study 131–3; and conductor 84–5, 132; definition of 83; as destructive aspect of groups 53; developmental 86; Nitsun on 88n3; pathological 84–5; and 'pro-group' 86
anxiety: and attachment theory 106, 116; causes of 76n1; in groups 81, 108, 112, 129, 130, 132, 133; and music performance 109–10, 145, 153; and Post-Traumatic Stress Disorder (PTSD) 129

APMT. *See* Association of Professional Music Therapists (APMT)
Argelander, H. 57
art therapy 17
Ashbach, C. 77n4
Association of Professional Music Therapists (APMT) 4
Association of Therapeutic Communities 19
assumptions 33. *See also* basic assumption theory
Athena 45
attachment theory: and anxiety 106, 116; attachment categories 105–6; Bowlby on 103–4; Bowlby's research 101–3; and creativity 110; and defences 106; and deficient early mothering 116; developmental pathways 104; vs. drive theory 104; and group analysis 103, 106–7; influence of, on group analysis 72; and interconnectedness 101–3; and relationships 104; role of early deprivation 103
attunement 39, 74, 107. *See also* affect attunement
authenticity, through group music therapy 7
authority: and conductor 48–9; as developmental task 32; as transferable 49
availability 107

Bacal, H. A. 74
Barenboim, Daniel x
Barnes, B. 64, 66
barometric event 35

Baron-Cohen, S. 95
Barwick, N. 31, 44
basic assumption theory: aggregation/ massification 88n2; and anti-groups 83; definition of 78; dependency 78, 80, 83; and exclusion dynamic 80, 81; fight-flight 78–9, 80, 83; grouping 88n2; and hierarchically structured groups 80; incohesion 82–3; me-ness 81–2, 88n2; oneness 81, 88n2; pairing 79, 80, 83
Bateson, G. 46
Beck, W. 57–8
Beecroft, Sue 16, 17
Behr, H. 47, 62, 66n4, 88, 140–1
Bennis, W. G. 35
Berg, D. N. 88n3
Bhaktin, M. 87
Bion, Wilfred: on basic assumptions 78; and basic assumption theory 10; on negative capability 76n1; source of basic assumptions 80; and Tavistock model 79; on valency 35; view of groups, vs. Foulkes' 79–80
Blunden, J. 135
Bollas, C. 34, 43, 54, 68, 92, 97
bonding capacity 84
boundaries: in case study 123; and conductor role 157–9; and principles of conduct 50–1
boundary incidents 30, 50
Bowlby, J. 72, 101–2, 103–4, 105, 117–18. *See also* attachment theory
British Journal of Music Therapy 141
British Journal of Psychotherapy 11
Britton, R. 44, 80
Brown, D. 33, 41, 51, 80, 87
Burruth, M. 37, 59

Cage, John 100
Cambridge Group Work 16, 17
CAMT. *See* Cognitive Analytic Music Therapy (CAMT)
Cano, D. H. 88n2
capitalist culture 23
case studies: boundaries 123; countertransference 123; of group music therapy 111–38; transference 123; of vitality affects 94–5
CAT. *See* Cognitive Analytic Therapy (CAT)
chain phenomena 34

change: ambivalence toward 111; as developmental task 32; pairing as defence against 79; in Western music 117
children: and attachment theory 102; music therapy for special needs 7–9
Clark, David 16, 17
clinical vignettes. *See* case studies
Cognitive Analytic Music Therapy (CAMT) 133–6
Cognitive Analytic Therapy (CAT) 134–5
coherence: definition of 31; and matrix 37; in time-limited groups 31–2
cohesion: and aggregation/massification 82; in case study 126–8; definition of 31; and empathy 73
collective unconscious 40
communication: autistic symptom 40–1; in case study 137; and complexity theory 87–8; and confrontation 61; as containment 69; and countertransference 57; and empathy 41; and exchange 46; facilitation of, as intervention 58–9; and forms of dialogue 41; levels of, in groups 40; monologue 41, 60; music as safe mode of 152; non-verbal 94–5, 97, 99, 130; resistance in 59–61; and resonance 39; and translation 41; turn-taking 60; and the unconscious 32–3; via music 116; in words and music 154. *See also* dialogue; exchange; language
community: Odell-Miller's experience of 19; responsibility of, for mental health 29
complexity theory 87–8
complex responsive processes 87
composition: of groups 30–1, 40. *See also* selection
Compton, S. J. 134, 135
conductor: and anti-groups 84–5, 132; and authority 48–9; in case study 126–8, 135; and containing 69; and countertransference 56–8; definition of 30, 48; as environmental mother 71; as father 49; as 'feminine' 53; Foulkes on 48; interventions by 53–8; and one-to-one attachment 52; and resistance 59–65; role of 157–9; roles of 48–9; and settings 49–50; silence of 53; and transference 50, 55–6. *See also* co-therapists; interventions

conflict 88n3
confrontation 61, 156
container: and containing 69; mother as 68; music as 100
containing: and anti-groups 86; of container 69; and countertransference 68; definition of 67; Foulkes on 68; and projective identification 67–8
containment: and anti-groups 83, 85; communication as 69; failure of 68
conversation. *See* communication
Cortesao, E. L. 86
co-therapists: from different disciplines 146; helpers/nurses 146–7; music therapist and trainee 143–4; music therapists 141–3; as parental couple 140–1, 148; trainees 144–6; and transference 148
co-therapy: case study of 141–3; Foulkes on 139–40; reasons for 140–1; and subgroups 147; supervision 143, 144, 145, 147–8
countertransference: in case study 123; and conductor 56–8; and containing 68; and experiential groups for students 159–61
creativity, and therapeutic process 113

Dalal, F. 33, 46, 87
Dang, J. C. 147
Darnley-Smith, R. 3, 4–5, 8
Davies, Alison 21, 141–3, 147–8
Davis, Graham 18, 19
defences: and attachment theory 106; basic assumptions as 78
dementia 94, 121–3
dependency 10, 61, 78, 80, 83
deprivation 103
Deri, S. 70
development, of groups 31–2
developmental pathways 104
de Waal, F. B. M. 74
dialectics 86
dialogue: forms of 41; and triadic mirroring 45–6. *See also* communication
Diel, P. 45
disavowals 33
discourse 41
diversity: and experiential groups for students 156–7; in groups 30–1; intolerance of 63, 66n4, 78–9
Down's Syndrome 137
drama therapy 17

dreams: Foulkes on 38; group dream 40
drive theory 104
drop-outs 64, 66n5, 112, 126
Duggan, C. 133
dynamic administration: boundaries 50–1; and conductor 49–52; selection of group members 51–2; settings 49–50, 50–1
dynamic matrix 36, 37, 153

Elias, Norbert 27, 28, 87
emotional contagion 74
empathic resonance 73, 74
empathy: and affect attunement 95–6; and communication 41; and mother–infant relationship 73–5; and touch 95
ending 64–5
engagement, as developmental task 32
environmental mother 70, 71
envy 82, 135
Eschen, Johannes 7
exchange: definition of 46; as non-verbal 47; as transformational 46; turn-taking 60. *See also* communication
exclusion: and basic assumptions 80; in case study 134; and experiential groups for students 156–7. *See also* scapegoating
experiential groups: and conductor role 157–9; countertransference 159–61; diversity and tolerance 156–7; and matrix 153; mirroring in 154–5; and projective identification 157; purpose of 150–1; and resonance 155–6; student training 149–62; and transference 157, 159–61
Ezriel, H. 79

facilitation, by conductor 53–4
false self 70, 71
fantasies 65
fascism 48
fight-flight 10, 78–9, 80, 83
figuration 28
focal conflict 60
foetal movements, and mother's voice 93–4
Fonagy, P. 116
Foulkes, S. H. ix–x; on amplification and condenser phenomenon 40; on conductor 48; on containment 68; on co-therapy 139–40; on

countertransference 57; on dreams 38; on free association 34; on group anxiety 108; on group as mother 67, 75; on group communication 40; on group matrix 38; on groups 133; on holistic approach 27–9; on interpretation 54, 55; on interventions 58; on introduction of new members 81; on matrix 36–7, 153; on mirroring 42, 154; model of three 44; on observer's role 44; as originator of group analysis 27; orthodox vs. radical 87; on patient as 'assistant therapist' 62; on psychoanalytic processes in groups 32; on resonance 38–9; on scapegoating 63; on selection 51; on socialisation 47; theories of, and group music therapy 10; on transference 34, 35, 55–6; on translation 41; view of groups, vs. Bion's 79–80. *See also* group analysis
foundation matrix 37, 153
free association 34, 159
Freud, S. 55, 67, 104
Fulbourn Hospital 12, 15, 16

Gahir, M. 135
Garland, C. 41
Gestalt psychology 27
Goldstein, Kurt 27, 87
Greenland, Sue 152
Grotjhan, M. 56
group, vs. individual, as false dichotomy 28
group analysis: and attachment theory 103, 106–7; core concepts of 29–32; Foulkes as originator of 27; mother–infant paradigm in 67; and music therapy xii; optimistic vs. pessimistic model of 79; and play 72; suitability for 51; vs. Tavistock model 88n1; vs. traditional psychoanalysis 27. *See also* Foulkes, S. H.
group-as-a-whole, and individual 152–3
group formation, parallels with mother–infant paradigm 71
grouping 88n2
group matrix. *See* matrix
group mind 38
group music therapy: Analytical Music Therapy (AMT) 4, 5–6; anti-group 131–3; and authenticity 7; case studies of 111–38; Cognitive Analytic Music Therapy (CAMT) 133–6; ending of 161–2; and Foulkes 10; Foulkes' influence on 10; historical perspective 3–11, 12–23; improvisation in 112–13; and John 10; for mothers and infants 124–6; and Nordoff and Robbins 7–8; and Odell-Miller 11; and Priestley 4–7; recent research on xii; silence in 6–7, 9, 155; and Streeter 9; and transference 11; and Woodcock 10–11. *See also* music therapy
group-object relations 84
groups: and anti-groups 53, 83–6; anxiety in 81, 108, 112, 129, 130, 132, 133; Bion vs. Foulkes' view of 79–80; coherence of 31; cohesion in 31; composition of 30–1, 40; development of 31–2, 161; diversity in 30–1; ending of 161–2; Foulkes on 133; free association 34; introduction of new members 52, 81, 111; and matrix 36–8; as mother 67, 75, 81; music in 101; Odell-Miller on experiences of 12–14; psychoanalytic processes in 32–5; size of 30; slow open 30, 31, 121; stranger group 30; tasks vs. stages 32; time-limited 30, 31–2, 65; transference in 34–5; as transitional object 77n4; Tuckman's group-stage summary 32; the unconscious in 32–3
guided facilitation 54
Guildhall School of Music and Drama 4, 5, 128
Guntrip, H. 76–7n3

Hall, T. W. 106
harmonising 95
Harris, T. 107
Harwood, I. 74
Hearst, L. 47, 88, 140–1
high secure hospital setting 133–6
Hinshelwood, R. 79
holding environment: absence of 82; analytic setting as 70–1; definition of 69; and false self 70; and withholding 71. *See also* mother–infant paradigm
holistic approach 27–9
Holmes, J. 102, 110, 116, 117
hope 79
Hopper, E. 35n1, 38, 51, 87, 88n2
Horwitz, L. 79
Hudson, Inge 16, 139, 140, 146, 147
Hutchinson, S. 49

idealisation 73
improvisation: and affect attunement 95; in case study 129–31, 132; and change 117; as expressive of group dynamics 9, 11, 130–1, 137–8, 155–6, 159–61; in group music therapy 112–13; and interconnectedness 118; lack of structure in 114–15; mirroring in 154–5; Odell-Miller on 12; and play 125; and relationships 152; and Western music 110–11
incohesion 82–3
independence 61
individual: vs. group, as false dichotomy 28; and group-as-a-whole 152–3; and matrix 37; as nodal point 36
individualism, and me-ness 82
individual therapy 30, 34
infancy: and empathy 73–4; exchange in 46; and mirroring 42; play in 70; separateness in 69–70, 96, 97; transitional object 70; transitional space 70. *See also* mother–infant paradigm; mother–infant relationship
inner child 154
Institute of Group Analysis 102
interconnectedness: and attachment theory 101–3; and experiential groups for students 151; and improvisation 118; and matrix 36–7; and musical experience 109; principle of 27–9; and resonance 155
inter-dependence 61
interdependence 28
interpretation: and anti-groups 84–5; Foulkes on 54, 55; as intervention 54–5; 'plunging' 54. *See also* translation
intersubjective theory 57
Intertherap 6, 7, 15. *See also* Priestley, Mary
interventions: in case study 126–8; countertransference 56–8; facilitation of communication as 58–9; guided facilitation 54; interpretation 54–5; maintenance 53; open facilitation 53; reasons for 58–65; for resistance 59–65; therapeutic 52–3; transference interpretation 55–6. *See also* conductor
intimacy, as developmental task 32
intolerance 63
intra-psychic processes, as non-verbal 136

Islam x
isolates 61–2, 66n4, 111, 113–14

James, C. D. 71
James, Colin 19
Jennings, Sue 16
John, David 10, 19, 21
Jones, Maxwell 16, 17
Joseph, B. 55
Journal of British Music Therapy 9, 10
Jung, C. 39, 40

Kernberg, O. 56
Klein, M. 103
Kohut, H. 73

Laing, R. D. 103
language: development of 91–2. *See also* communication
Lavie, J. 29, 81
Lawrence, W. G. 82
learning, in mother–infant dyad 91
learning disabilities 136–8
Levine, S. 112–13, 115, 147
Lewin, K. 66
Lieberman, M. A. 60
linking 84
Lintott, Bill 155, 158
location: and anti-groups 85; as aspect of group mind 38
loss 80

maintenance 53
Malan, D. 55
malignant mirroring 44, 45, 61, 69
Malinowski, B. 59
Marrone, M. 101, 107
Marsh, L. C. 29
matrix: definition of 36; dynamic matrix 36, 153; and experiential groups 153; foundation matrix 37, 153; group matrix 38; personal group matrix 36, 153; resistance to joining 61–3; and resonance 39, 155
McGee, T. 148
Mead, G. H. 87
Medusa 45
Meltzer, D. 55
me-ness 81–2, 88n2
mental health: community's responsibility for 29; and mother–infant relationship 124

mental illness, and early deprivation 103
Merleau-Ponty, M. 47
mimetic engulfment 43
mirroring: and affect-sharing 74; definition of 42; and dialogue 45–6; and empathy 73; and experiential groups for students 154–5; in improvisation 154–5; and infancy 42; malignant mirroring 44, 45, 61, 69; negative 43–4; and projective identification 42–3; triadic 44–6
mirror neurons 43, 74, 75
misattunement 107
mistrust 75–6
Mitchell, Sydney 3
model of three 44
models. *See* working models
monitoring 159–61
monologue 41, 60. *See also* communication
Morgan, G. 86
mother–infant paradigm: containing 67–8; and empathy 75; in group analysis 67; holding 69; object vs. environmental mother 70; parallels with group formation 71. *See also* infancy
mother–infant relationship: and affect attunement 95–7, 117; and language development 91–2; learning in 91; and mental health 124; and mother's voice 93–4; overview of 91–2; and sensitive responsiveness 104–6; sonic imagery in 92; stimulation in 92; transitional objects 98; vitality affects 92–5
mothers: elementary vs. transformational 76; frightening or deficient 75–6, 116; groups as 67, 75, 81; idealisation of 76
movement, as vitality affect 93
music: Barenboim on x; communication via 116; and emotional experience 100; as escape from narcissism 117; and interconnectedness 109; psychoanalytic view of 10; as safe communication mode 152; as social 100; Steiner on xiii; as structural frame 100; as therapeutic medium 100–1; tradition of, to promote health x; Western 110–11, 117
music performance, anxiety regarding 109–10, 145, 153
music therapy: and affect attunement 97; and group analysis xii; origins of x; and psychoanalysis 10; Streeter on approaches to 9; talking vs. playing

music in 11; and transitional space 99; and vitality affects 96, 97. *See also* group music therapy

narcissism: and anti-groups 85; and monologue 41; music as escape from 117; and negative mirroring 43–4
Nava, A. S. 74
negative capability 76n1
negative mirroring 43–4. *See also* mirroring
negative transference 7, 157
Nieman, Alfred 5, 12, 13, 15
Nitsun, M.: on anti-group 83, 84, 85, 88n3; on anti-group and 'pro-group' 86; on Foulkes 66n1; on group development 71; on mirroring 43; on play 86; on primal scene 80–1. *See also* anti-group
nodal point, individual as 36
Nordoff, Paul 7–8

object mother 70
object relations theory 57, 83, 104
observer, role of 44
occupational therapy 15
Odell-Miller, Helen: on group experiences 12–14; on improvisation 12; interview with 12–24; and Priestley 15; role of, in origins of group music therapy 11
Oedipal situation 45, 80–1, 135
Ogden, T. H. 86
Oldfield, Amelia 22
omnipotence 65, 78
oneness 81, 88n2
open facilitation 53
Orange, D. M. 75
Ormont, L. R. 61, 62
Ornstein, P. 74

Padel, J. 46
pairing 10, 79, 80, 83
passion for proximity 84
Patey, H. 3, 4–5, 8
patients: case studies of 111–38; and group composition 51–2; isolates 61–2; music therapy's functions for 9; and one-to-one attachment 52; as therapists in group therapy 58, 62
Pavlicevic, M. 100
Pegasus 45
Perseus 44–5
personal group matrix 36, 153

personification 35
phatic communion 59
Pickett, Maggie 13
Pines, M.: on conductor 49; on discourse 41; on group as mother 67; on group as selfobject 73; on group composition 51; on group development 32; on interpretation 54; on mirroring 42; on resistant conversations 59; on transference 35; on triadic mirroring 44–6
play 70, 72, 86, 115, 125
plunging interpretation 54
Post-Traumatic Stress Disorder (PTSD), in case study 128–31
Powell, A. 37, 157
power relations 87
Preston, S. D. 74
Priestley, Mary 4–7, 15, 101. *See also* Analytical Music Therapy (AMT)
primal scene 80–1
primitive group mentality 78, 79, 85
Prodgers, A. 56–7, 66n3, 75, 76
projective identification: and anti-groups 83; and containing 67–8; and countertransference 57, 58; as destructive force 69; and experiential groups for students 157; and mirroring 42–3; and transference 35
prosody 94
Psychiatric Interest Group 19
psychoanalysis: and music therapy 10; traditional, vs. group model 27
psychopathology 86
PTSD. *See* Post-Traumatic Stress Disorder (PTSD)

Qinodoz, Danielle 121

reenactments 57
regression: and basic assumptions 79; caused by ending 64–5; and dependency 80
relationships: and attachment theory 104; and improvisation 152. *See also* attachment theory; mother–infant relationship
resistance: to change 117; conductor's interventions for 59–65; and drop-outs 64; to ending 64–5; and free association 34; against independence 61; to integrating difference 63; to matrix 61–3; silence as 64

resonance: amplification and condenser phenomenon 40; and communication 39; and countertransference 57; definition of 38–9, 155; and experiential groups for students 155–6; and interconnectedness 155; and matrix 155; in mother–infant dyad 95–6; and social bonding 39
Richards, Eleanor 141–3, 147–8
Robbins, Clive 7–8
Roberts, J. 38, 59, 73, 133
Roberts, Vega 20
Roehampton Institute 20, 21
Rogers, C. 58, 68
Rose, Chris 150, 154

scapegoating 38, 63, 69, 134. *See also* exclusion
scenic understanding 57–8
Schermer, V. L. 43, 77n4
Schlachet, P. 72
Schlapobersky, J. 32, 41, 51, 58, 161
Scholz, R. 37
Schuman, B. J. 148
Segal, H. 68
Segalla, R. 75
selection: and anti-groups 84; criteria for 51–2; Foulkes on 51; of group members 51–2; and new members 52, 81, 111
selfobjects 73–4
self-psychology: and countertransference 57; and empathy 73
sensitive responsiveness 104–6
settings: in case study 115; challenges to 50–1; of group therapy 49–50; high secure hospital 133–6; and table as transitional object 66n2
Sharpe, Meg 19
Shepard, H. A. 35
Sherbourne, Veronica 15–16
silence: in case study 132; of conductor 53; and connectedness 9; in group music therapy 6–7, 155; and incohesion 82; as resistance 64
size, of groups 30
Sklar, John 19
Sleight, V. 134
slow open groups 30, 31, 121
Smith, K. K. 88n3
social bonding 39
social defences 33
socialisation 47
social matrix 37

social unconscious 87
socio-cultural constructs 33
sonic imagery 92
Spiers, Ronald 16
splitting 76
Stacey, R. 87, 88, 88n4
staff support groups 17
St. Bernard's Hospital 4
Steele, Pamela 20
Stein, A. 117
Steiner, George xiii, 152
Stern, D.: on affect attunement 74, 96; on infant language 47; on misattunement 107; on mother–infant relationship 91; on stimulus 92; on vitality affects 93–4
stimulation 92, 94
Storr, A. 117
storytelling, and music therapy 8–9
stranger group 30
Streeter, Elaine 9, 20, 21, 159
structural oppression 33
student training: and co-therapy 143–6; experiential groups 149–62; Odell-Miller on 21–3
Sunfield House 8
supervision: in co-therapy 143, 144, 145, 147–8; in student training 22
Syminton, Neville 18
system-as-a-whole 27–8
systems theory 86–7

Tavistock model 79–80, 88n1
termination, as developmental task 32
therapist: as authority 49; as detached 79, 80; and empathic resonance 74; and holding environment 70–1; patient as, in group therapy 58, 62; and transference 34. *See also* conductor; co-therapists
Thygesen, B. 39
time-limited groups 30, 31–2, 65
Toder, M. 43
tonality 117
touch 95
Towse, Esme 11
training courses. *See* student training
transference: in case study 123; and conductor 50; co-therapists 148; definition of 11; and experiential groups for students 157, 159–61; Foulkes on 55–6; and group music therapy 11; in groups 34–5; negative 75, 157; and personification 35; whole object vs. part object 34

transference interpretation 55–6
transformation: and anti-groups 86; empathy's role in 73; and exchange 46
transitional object 66n2, 70, 77n4, 98–9
transitional space 70, 72, 86, 99
translation 41, 55. *See also* interpretation
trauma 103, 128–31
Trevarthen, C. 54
triadic mirroring 44–6. *See also* mirroring
Tubert-Oklander, J. 41
Tuckman, B. 32
turn-taking 60
twinship 73

the unconscious: collective unconscious 40; and countertransference 56–7; dual model of 33; in groups 32–3; social 32–3, 87

valency 35, 79
Vella, N. 88n4
vitality affects: and affect attunement 96; clinical vignette 94–5; definition of 92–3; and mother–infant relationship 93–4; and music therapy 96, 97
Vygotsky, L. 87

Wallin, D. 114
Walrond-Skinner, S. 140
Warley Hospital 10
Warlingham Park Hospital 3
Weinberg, H. 38, 43
Whitaker, D. S. 60
Wigram, Tony 14–15
Winnicott, D. W.: on conductor as environmental mother 71; and Guntrip 76–7n3; on holding environment 69; on mother–infant relationship 123; on play 70, 71–2; on transitional object 98
witnessing 58. *See also* triadic mirroring
Wolf, E. S. 74
Woodcock, John 10–11, 19
Wooster, G. 42, 45
work group 78
working models 105, 107–8, 112, 117–18
Wright, K. 95, 97, 98, 99

Yogev, H. 71, 75

Zinkin, L.: on exchange 46; on group matrix 37; on malignant mirroring 44; and mirroring 42; on primordial level in groups 40; on vitality affects 92

eBooks
from Taylor & Francis

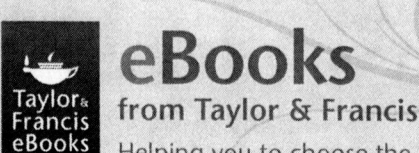

Helping you to choose the right eBooks for your Library

Add to your library's digital collection today with Taylor & Francis eBooks. We have over 45,000 eBooks in the Humanities, Social Sciences, Behavioural Sciences, Built Environment and Law, from leading imprints, including Routledge, Focal Press and Psychology Press.

Choose from a range of subject packages or create your own!

Benefits for you
- Free MARC records
- COUNTER-compliant usage statistics
- Flexible purchase and pricing options
- 70% approx of our eBooks are now DRM-free.

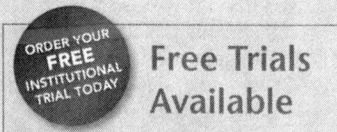

Free Trials Available

We offer free trials to qualifying academic, corporate and government customers.

ORDER YOUR FREE INSTITUTIONAL TRIAL TODAY

Benefits for your user
- Off-site, anytime access via Athens or referring URL
- Print or copy pages or chapters
- Full content search
- Bookmark, highlight and annotate text
- Access to thousands of pages of quality research at the click of a button.

eCollections

Choose from 20 different subject eCollections, including:

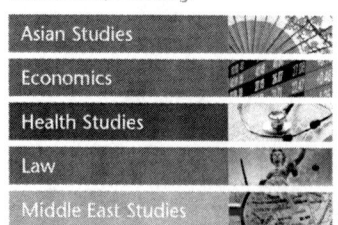

- Asian Studies
- Economics
- Health Studies
- Law
- Middle East Studies

eFocus

We have 16 cutting-edge interdisciplinary collections, including:

- Development Studies
- The Environment
- Islam
- Korea
- Urban Studies

For more information, pricing enquiries or to order a free trial, please contact your local sales team:

UK/Rest of World: **online.sales@tandf.co.uk**
USA/Canada/Latin America: **e-reference@taylorandfrancis.com**
East/Southeast Asia: **martin.jack@tandf.com.sg**
India: **journalsales@tandfindia.com**

www.tandfebooks.com